W9-CKB-237

ENCYCLOPEDIA OF
FAMILY HEALTH

ENCYCLOPEDIA OF

FAMILY HEALTH

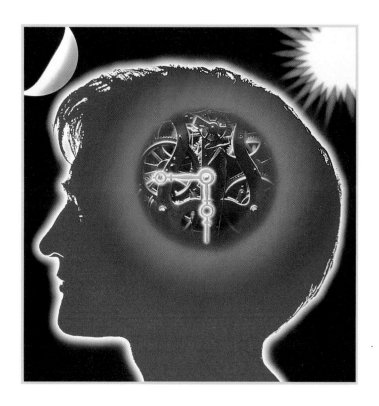

CONSULTANT
DAVID B. JACOBY, MD
JOHNS HOPKINS SCHOOL OF MEDICINE

VOLUME
2

BANDAGES—CARPAL TUNNEL SYNDROME

MARSHALL CAVENDISH
NEW YORK · LONDON · TORONTO · SYDNEY

Marshall Cavendish Corporation

99 White Plains Road

Tarrytown, New York 10591-9001

© Marshall Cavendish Corporation, 1998

© Marshall Cavendish Limited 1998, 1991, 1988, 1986, 1983, 1982, 1971

Update by Brown Partworks

The material in this set was first published in the English language by

Marshall Cavendish Limited of 119 Wardour Street, London W1V 3TD, England.

Printed and bound in Italy

Library of Congress Cataloging-in-Publication Data

Encyclopedia of family health
17v. cm.
Includes index
1. Medicine, Popular-Encyclopedias. 2. Health-Encyclopedias. I. Marshall Cavendish Corporation.
RC81.A2M336 1998   96-49537
610'.3-dc21   CIP
ISBN 0-7614-0625-5 (set)
ISBN 0-7614-0627-1 (v.2)

INTRODUCTION

We Americans live under a constant bombardment of information (and misinformation) about the latest supposed threats to our health. We are taught to believe that disease is the result of not taking care of ourselves. Death becomes optional. Preventive medicine becomes a moral crusade, illness the punishment for the foolish excesses of the American lifestyle. It is not the intent of the authors of this encyclopedia to contribute to this atmosphere. While it is undoubtedly true that Americans could improve their health by smoking less, exercising more, and controlling their weight, this is already widely understood.

As Mencken put it, "It is not the aim of medicine to make men virtuous. The physician should not preach salvation, he should offer absolution." The aims of this encyclopedia are to present a summary of human biology, anatomy, and physiology, to outline the more common diseases, and to discuss, in a general way, the diagnosis and treatment of these diseases. This is not a do-it-yourself book. It will not be possible to treat most conditions based on the information presented here. But it will be possible to understand most diseases and their treatments. Informed in this way, you will be able to discuss your condition and its treatment with your physician. It is also hoped that this will alleviate some of the fears associated with diseases, doctors, and hospitals.

The authors of this encyclopedia have also attempted to present, in an open-minded way, alternative therapies. There is undoubtedly value to some of these. However, when dealing with serious diseases, they should not be viewed as a substitute for conventional treatment. The reason that conventional treatment is accepted is that it has been systematically tested, and because scientific evidence backs it up. It would be a tragedy to miss the opportunity for effective treatment while pursuing an ineffective alternative therapy.

Finally, it should be remembered that the word *doctor* is originally from the Latin word for "teacher." Applied to medicine, this should remind us that the doctor's duty is not only to diagnose and treat disease, but to help the patient to understand. If this encyclopedia can aid in this process, its authors will be gratified.

DAVID B. JACOBY, MD
JOHNS HOPKINS SCHOOL OF MEDICINE

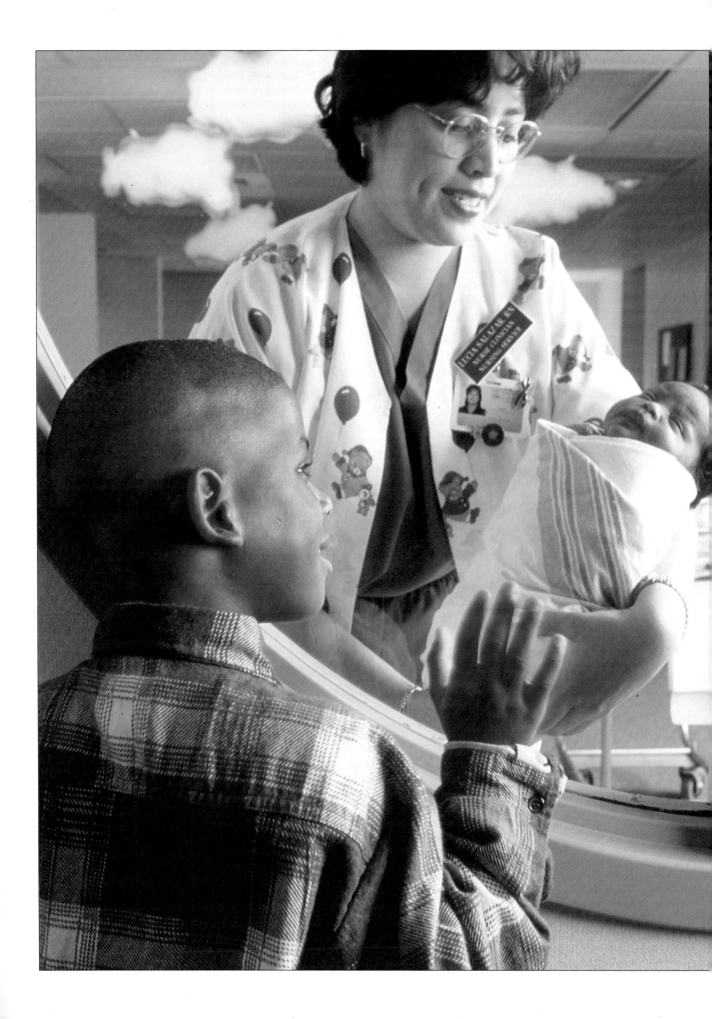

CONTENTS

Bandages

Bandaging is a vital part of first aid, and it is necessary in many emergencies. But there are several different types of bandage, so it is essential to know which type to choose and exactly how to use it for a particular purpose.

Q Does it matter if I get my bandage wet?

A A bandage covering a recent wound or one where there is discharge from the skin should not be allowed to get wet, because germs could be washed through to the inner dressing. In most other circumstances, it does not matter. However, a wet bandage will be uncomfortable to wear and may become loose as it dries, so wet bandages are best replaced with dry ones.

Q I am restocking my medicine chest. Which types of bandages should I buy?

A It is best to have a range of sizes and types on hand. You should include small, medium, and large wound dressings; 1 in (2.5 cm), 2 in (5 cm), and 3 in (7.5 cm) bandages; one or two crepe bandages; a triangular bandage to use as a sling; and a packet of Band-Aids. You may also like to include a tubular gauze finger bandage. Remember to carry out a regular check on the contents of your medicine chest and replace any items that have been used.

Q Can bandages irritate the skin or cause allergies?

A Allergies to cloth bandages are extremely rare. The heavy elastic bandages that are often used to treat severe leg ulcers do contain rubber, however, and this could possibly cause an allergic reaction.

Q I'm afraid that in a real emergency I will forget how to do a bandage properly. Do you have any tips?

A The main thing is to act quickly and not to panic. It doesn't matter if you don't get the bandage exactly right, because it can always be redone properly later. What is important in most cases is to stop the bleeding—by bandaging firmly or, at least, pressing on the wound. If you don't have any proper bandages available, improvise with whatever is available.

There are a number of different types of bandages, each used for a specific type of injury. Typical uses include:
- holding a dressing in position over a wound, and adding to the protection provided by the dressing
- preventing movement of an injured part of the body
- providing direct pressure to stop or control bleeding
- providing additional support to strengthen a weakened joint, for

A sling is a hanging bandage used to provide support for an injured limb. In an emergency, improvise one from a scarf.

example, a knee joint after injury
- applying pressure to reduce swelling
- holding a splint in position
- assisting in the carrying of a badly injured person

Types of bandage

Bandages can be made from any clothlike substance, including calico, linen, cotton, gauze, muslin, crepe, flannel, and even paper. They are available in a variety of shapes and sizes and are designed to be employed for a wide range of uses.

The triangular bandage is made by cutting a square of linen or calico into two triangles with sides at least one yard

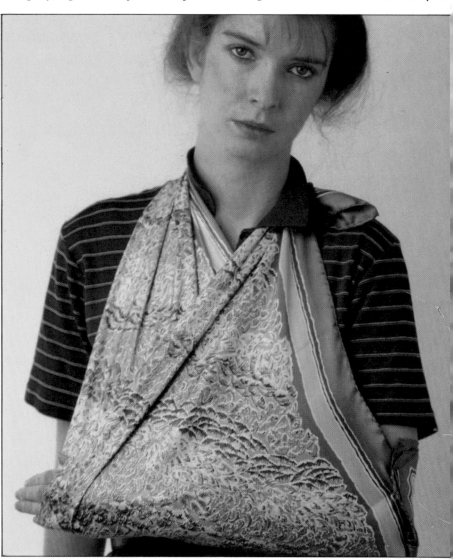

(1 m) long. Although using it requires skill, and it can sometimes be difficult to knot safely, the triangular bandage can be used in many ways. As a whole cloth, it can hold a large dressing in position or be made into a sling. It can also be folded to make either a broad or a narrow bandage. When it is folded into a ring shape, it forms an excellent pressure pad that can be used to control bleeding, or for protecting a broken or fractured bone from accidental bangs and knocks that may occur.

The roller bandage is a roll of open-weave cloth such as cotton, muslin, crepe, flannel, or special paper. It is cheap to buy and comes in various widths for different parts of the body. The roller bandage is nonstretch and can therefore almost never be fixed too tightly. This type of bandage can be difficult to apply, however, because it does not mold firmly to the contours of the body in the same way that a stretch bandage does. More skill and practice are therefore required to apply it well.

The basic application technique is to use the left hand firmly, but gently, to support and guide the injured part of the body, while the right hand holds the bandage, letting it out to cover the wound. It should be applied securely, with each new turn covering about two-thirds of the previous turn.

The crepe bandage is probably the most popular bandage. Woven to have elastic strength, it is stretchy enough to cling firmly to uneven body surfaces and provide a measure of firm support. It can be used in almost every circumstance, and very little skill is required to apply it correctly. If this kind of bandage is fixed too tightly, however, it can be very dangerous, because it has enough strength to cut off the blood supply.

The tubular bandage is a long tube of gauze that is applied in layers to a finger or a limb, using a special applicator. The size of the applicator varies according to the particular part of the body for which it is designed to be used.

Fixing a bandage

Bandages must be applied firmly to be effective. Any bandage that is applied too tightly and left on for any length of time may interfere with the blood circulation and lead first to the permanent damage of an area, and then possibly to the development of gangrene (see Gangrene) if the bandage is not loosened in time.

A simple test for good circulation in a bandaged limb is to press on any nail. It should immediately turn white. When the pressure is removed, the blood should return within two seconds, making the nail appear naturally pink again. If this

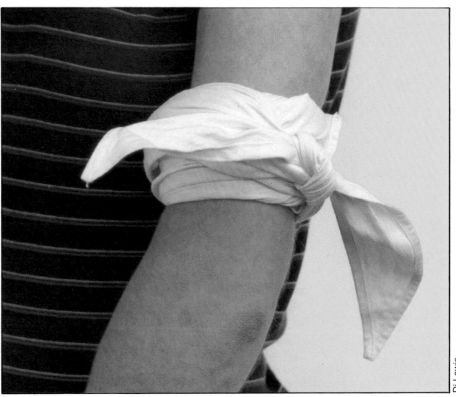

A bandage that is too tight cuts off circulation, producing swelling and pain. The limb loses its pulse, becomes numb or tingly, and shows a whitish tinge.

Di Lewis

does not happen, loosen the bandage at once and test again in the same manner.

Bandages can be fixed in a number of ways. If you secure them by tying a knot, it is best to use a reef knot. Since this is a flat knot, it will not rub the injured part of the body under the bandage, which would cause irritation or even more pain for the patient.

Small safety pins lie flat and are ideal for fixing stretch bandages. They should be passed through the two outermost layers of the fabric.

Adhesive tape is often sufficient to hold bandages that will not get a lot of wear and scuffing. If a bandage is likely to be rubbed so much that it could become loose, a small stretch bandage clip can be used as well.

When not to bandage

Never use a bandage to completely cover an area that requires regular observation. When a limb is broken or a person is seriously injured and an ambulance has been called, it is best to leave the job of bandaging the victim to the ambulance staff or a doctor. Concentrate all your efforts on comforting the patient and seeing that he or she is settled as comfortably as possible.

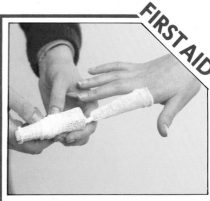

FIRST AID

Using a tubular bandage

Applying to the finger

1 Cut a piece of bandage of sufficient length from the pack and load it onto the applicator. Slip the applicator over the injured finger, then slip off the starting end of the bandage, holding it at the base of the finger if necessary.
2 Withdraw the applicator, letting the bandage slip off the end. When the applicator is clear of the finger, twist it one half turn.
3 Push another layer of bandage down in the same way, and repeat the process. Repeat until there are as many layers as needed. Finally, fix the bandage at the base of the finger with a ring of adhesive tape.

Using a triangular bandage

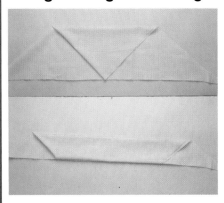

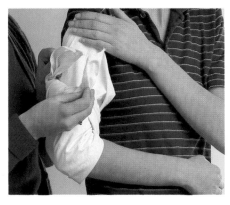

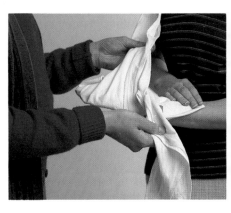

Making a broad or narrow bandage

1 Lay the triangular bandage on a flat surface, with the point of the bandage facing away from you.

2 To make a BROAD bandage, bring the point down to meet the middle of the base, then fold once again. To make a NARROW bandage, fold the broad bandage one more time. Smooth out any creases, and then fold lengthways for easy storage.

Making an elbow bandage

1 With the elbow bent, place the point of the bandage on the outer part of the upper arm, with the base across the underside of the forearm.

2 Cross the ends in front of the elbow, bring them back around the arm, and tie above the joint. Finally bring the flap formed by the point back over the knot, and fasten with a safety pin.

Making a hand bandage

1 Place the palm of the hand on the bandage, and bring the point of the bandage over toward the base.

2 Take the ends of the bandage and cross them around the wrist. Tie a reef knot over the point where the bandage lies on the back of the wrist.

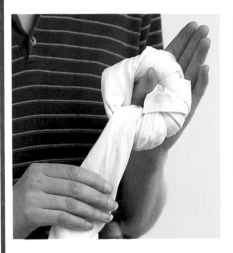

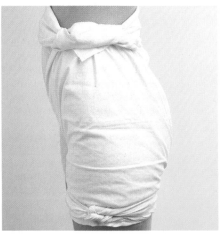

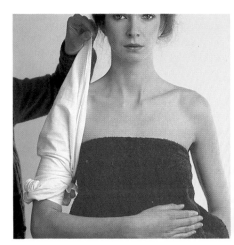

Making a ring pad

1 Make a narrow bandage and pass it loosely around the fingers of the left hand. Hold the formed circle and slip the bandage end through the loop.

2 Keep wrapping the loose end through the loop until it is all used and you have made a tight ring.

Making a hip bandage

1 Use two triangular bandages. First make a narrow bandage. Place it around the waist like a belt, tying a reef knot on the injured side. Next place the point of the second triangular bandage under the knot, and fold a hem along the base of the second bandage.

2 Holding the two ends of the hemmed base, take them around the thigh and buttock to the outer side, tying with a reef knot. Finally bring the point of the bandage down and secure the bandage with a safety pin.

Making a shoulder bandage

1 Fold a 1 in (2.5 cm) hem along the base of a triangular bandage. Position it on the arm so that the point of the bandage reaches the level of the ear.

2 Take the hem around the arm and cross the ends over. Bring them back to the outside and tie with a reef knot. Finally apply an arm sling, securing the point of the bandage to the sling with a safety pin.

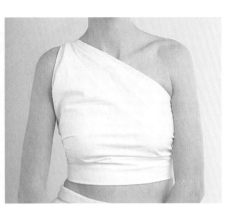

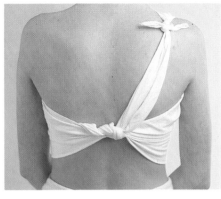

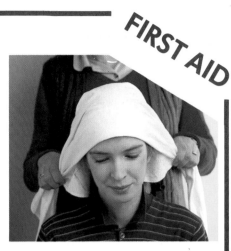

Making a chest bandage

1 Place the bandage over the front of the chest so that the point passes over one shoulder and the base lies across the chest.

2 Bring the two ends of the base around to the back and tie together. Bring the long end up to meet the point and secure it by tying a reef knot at the shoulder.

Making a head bandage

1 Hold both ends of the base of the triangular bandage. Fold a 1 in (2.5 cm) hem along that side. Place the hem on the forehead just above the eyebrows. The point should drop over the back of the patient's head.
2 Bring the ends around behind the head, crossing them firmly at the back of the neck. Bring the ends forward again, and tie with a reef knot over the forehead. Finally bring the point up over the crossed ends, and pin to the bandage on the top of the head.

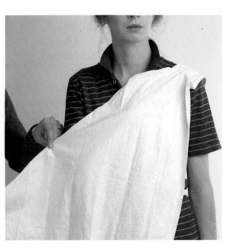

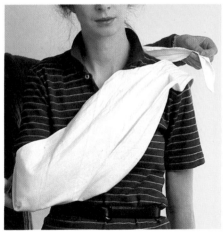

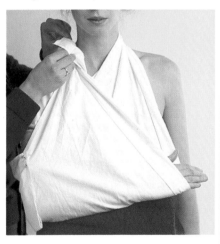

Making a triangular sling

1 The triangular sling is ideal for supporting an injured hand or forearm comfortably in a well-raised position. Place the injured arm or hand across the chest at the level of the opposite shoulder, and support it gently. Then place the open triangular bandage over the injured arm with the point about 6–9 in (15–23 cm) higher than the uninjured shoulder.

2 Gently ease the base area of the bandage under the injured arm, bringing one end around the back and up in front of the uninjured shoulder.
3 Tie a reef knot in the hollow under the collarbone and tuck the end of the bandage neatly in between the loose folds at the elbow. Secure the bandage with a safety pin.

Making a simple arm sling

1 The arm sling carries the weight of an injured arm, and it is the simplest sling to make. Place the injured arm at a level where the hand is just higher than the elbow. Pass an open triangular bandage between the chest and the arm, taking the point over the shoulder on the uninjured side.
2 Bring the lower end of the bandage up over the forearm to meet the point, and tie a knot over the natural hollow just above the collarbone. Pin the loose end of the bandage at the elbow.

Q Is there any rule about how long you can leave a bandage on before you have to change it?

A Bandages need changing when they become stained with discharge, dirty from general use, or loose from wear and movement. Stretch bandages compressing the limb beneath stretch quickly and need to be changed and reapplied daily. Roller bandages covering a dressing need only be changed when the dressing itself has to be replaced. But this will vary according to the instructions of the doctor or nurse, and in some cases patients are asked to leave bandages completely alone, no matter how soiled or dirty looking they may become.

Q How will I be able to tell if a bandage has become too tight as the result of swelling underneath it?

A Most injuries cause some degree of swelling as part of the healing process, and all bandages should therefore be checked at regular intervals. If a bandage feels too tight, there is swelling above and below it, or the area below it is painful, numb, blue, or white, the bandage could be blocking the circulation and doing more harm than good. Loosening the bandage will produce an immediate relief of symptoms, but if you are at all concerned, get a doctor's advice immediately.

Q What can be used to replace proper bandages in an emergency?

A Almost any material can be used as a temporary bandage. Cotton strips torn from skirts and dresses are ideal. Even ties, scarves, and belts can make good bandages. Panty hose or stockings have sufficient give in them to act as stretch bandages, and they provide extra compression. It is always better to improvise a bandage by using whatever material is available than to delay treating an injury. If the dressing covering an injury is sterile, the bandage need not be.

Using a roller bandage

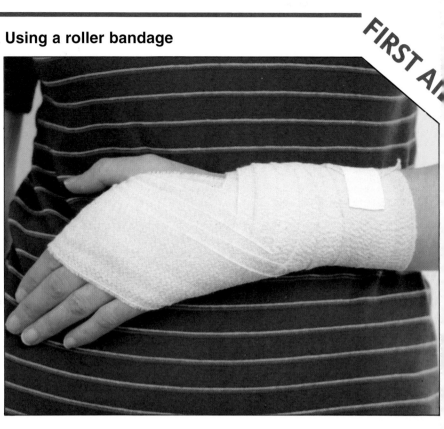

Applying to the hand
Use a 2 in (5 cm) wide bandage. Start from the wrist, make one turn, and secure the starting end of the bandage underneath. Pass the bandage over the back of the hand, around the little finger, and across the palm, leaving the thumb free. Finally bring the roll back to the wrist to finish off the bandage with a straight turn.

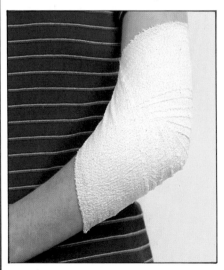

Applying to the elbow
1 With the elbow in a comfortable position, place the loose end of the bandage over the elbow crease. Take the first turn right around the joint itself.
2 Make further turns above and below the original turns in a figure eight, until sufficient area is covered.

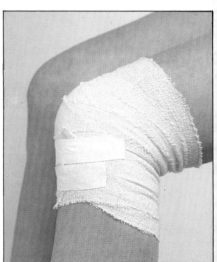

Applying to the knee
The technique is similar to bandaging the elbow. Make sure the knee is in a comfortable position. Starting at the back, take one straight turn over the joint, then bandage in a figure eight above and below, making sure you finish above the knee.

Barbiturates

Barbiturates are best known for their use as sleeping pills, but other drugs have now largely replaced them.

Q Is it really dangerous to take barbiturates when you are taking other drugs as well?

A Because of their strong effect on the liver, barbiturates interact badly with certain other drugs. Among these are anticoagulants, steroids (including the contraceptive pill), and some antidepressants. If you have been prescribed a barbiturate, and there is any chance that your doctor is not aware of other current drug treatment you are receiving, you should certainly tell him or her to insure there is no adverse reaction.

Q Is it safe to mix alcohol and barbiturates?

A Definitely not. The combination has a strong sedative effect, which could have fatal results if a person tries to drive a car in this state. Also the mixture of barbiturates and alcohol causes depression.

Q I have heard that a person taking sleeping pills may sometimes reach out in a dazed state at night for the bottle of pills and take additional doses. Is this just a way of explaining away a suicide attempt or can it really happen?

A The clinical term used to describe this is *drug automatism*, and it is possible for accidental overdoses to be taken in this way. Someone suffering from insomnia may wish to take more tablets in the night and, being already partially sedated, may accidentally take too many. This is why sleeping pills should never be left beside the bed at night.

Q Why are barbiturates not prescribed for a patient who is suffering from insomnia and who is in considerable pain at the same time?

A Barbiturates will not induce sleep when insomnia is due to pain. Instead they will make the patient restless and confused. An adequate painkiller, possibly supported by a safe sedative, is the answer in this case.

Barbiturates are usually divided into four groups, according to the strength and duration of their effect, i.e. long-acting, medium-acting, short-acting, and ultra-short-acting. They include phenobarbital, which is used as a sedative and antiepileptic (or anticonvulsant), and amylobarbital, which is used as a sedative. They are both long-acting. Quinalbarbital, which is short-acting, is used as a hypnotic, while thiopental (pentothal), an ultrashort-acting barbiturate, is used in anesthesia. Today, however, other drugs tend to be used instead.

Drawbacks

Barbiturates are depressants. Their strongest effect is on the central nervous

Barbiturates are still responsible for many cases of drug overdose among addicts and for many attempted suicides.

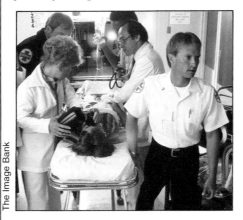

The Image Bank

system. They reduce the activity of nerve cells (or neurons), and the nerve centers of the brain that control consciousness and mental activity are affected first.

Two important brain centers affected are the respiratory and vasomotor centers. The respiratory center controls the rate of breathing, which is slowed down by barbiturates. Their effect on the vasomotor center is to reduce blood pressure.

Barbiturates also lower the body temperature and may lead to hypothermia (an excessively low body temperature), particularly in the elderly. They have a strong effect on the liver, speeding up its processes. This means that they can often interact badly if taken with other drugs.

Among other drawbacks, barbiturates can cause skin rashes and lead to mental confusion and fainting in the elderly. Patients taking them should not operate machinery or drive vehicles.

But the major disadvantage of barbiturates is that they result in dependence and addiction. Users also need to increase their dosage to achieve the same effect.

The results of overuse can be poor muscle coordination, difficulties with speech, and confused thinking. If the drugs are given up abruptly, there are unpleasant withdrawal symptoms that resemble those of alcohol withdrawal— restlessness, sleep disturbance, sweating, delirium, hallucinations, and convulsions.

Today other drugs are usually preferred, and barbiturates are used only as short-acting anesthetics, anticonvulsants, and for severe insomnia.

Treating an overdose

Signs of an overdose
A person who has taken a barbiturate overdose will become drowsy and then unconscious. The pupils of the eyes will dilate, and breathing may become dangerously slow. An overdose can poison the heart muscle, affecting the heartbeat, and dilate (widen) blood vessels, causing blood pressure to fall drastically. Blisters may appear.

Immediate help
Anyone discovering a person who has taken an overdose should summon professional help immediately. Call an ambulance, because a hospital emergency room is the best place for the patient's condition to be assessed.

Make sure that any pill bottles found near the person are given to the hospital to help identify the drug. In the hospital, a stomach pump may be used to wash out any remains of the drug. Some poisons can be removed by placing the patient on a kidney dialysis machine. In other cases, supportive therapy while the patient's system eliminates the drug is sufficient.

First aid
While you are waiting for help to arrive, make sure that the patient's nose and mouth are clear and that breathing is not obstructed. Lay the patient on his or her side to prevent vomit from being inhaled.

Barium liquids

Q My doctor says I need a barium meal. What does it taste like and will it hurt?

A The barium meal is made up of barium sulfate, which is chalky but not hard to swallow. It is a little like drinking liquid plaster. Often it is taken with a carbonated drink or sweetened and flavored in order to make it more palatable. Once the barium meal has been swallowed, it is impossible to feel it, and it causes no pain.

Q How long will it take for the barium meal to pass right through my system?

A On average it takes about 48 hours, but you may find that your feces are chalky for up to a week. The barium meal is likely to make you constipated, so you will probably be given a laxative to take after the treatment.

Q Will I have to stay in the hospital overnight?

A It will depend on whether the barium meal is to be combined with any other test and on what, if anything, is wrong, but the procedure can usually be carried out in one day. Sometimes patients are given a barium meal to take at home first thing in the morning, then asked to spend the day in the hospital for X rays.

Q Can I eat any food while the barium is inside me?

A The doctor will advise you to have a light supper, then nothing to eat on the day of the test, so that there is no chance of the barium being mixed with food.

Q My doctor suggested a barium meal to check for a peptic ulcer, but she hasn't ordered one yet. Shouldn't this be done right away?

A Barium meals are only necessary if there is substantial doubt about the presence of an ulcer due to lack of or conflicting symptoms. A very small ulcer may not show up in a barium X ray, in any event.

A barium meal is a dose of barium sulfate, the white, chalky substance that blocks X rays. This makes it possible for doctors to use X rays to take pictures of the alimentary canal for close examination.

The only parts of the body that show up on an X ray (see X rays) are those that block the passage of the rays, such as bones. The rays penetrate all softer parts, including skin, fat, and muscle. So if a doctor suspects that there is something wrong with a patient's intestine—for example, an ulcer, hernia, or tumor—an ordinary X-ray examination will produce only a fuzzy, indistinct picture.

Yet X rays remain one of the best ways of understanding what is happening inside the human body, especially when the precise source of a problem has not yet been identified.

Barium meal
A patient who is suspected of having an intestinal problem will be given a barium meal before the X ray. A barium meal is nothing like an ordinary meal: it is simply a cupful or so of a white, chalky substance called barium sulfate, which is completely insoluble and has the ability, just like bones, to block X rays.

On its own, barium sulfate is a tasteless, white, chalky powder that is completely harmless. This powder is either mixed with water to form a thick paste and swallowed, or a spoonful of the paste may be taken with a carbonated drink to make it more palatable. Other substances may be added to improve its coating powers and reduce foaming. Because barium sulfate is impossible to digest, there is no chance of it causing problems by getting into other parts of the body.

The barium sulfate mixture clings to the wall of the esophagus, stomach, and bowel, and shows up on an X ray as a dense, white outline. If there are any ulcers (lesions in the mucous membrane) present, they can be clearly seen, because the barium will travel into them and show up as projections extending out beyond the normal edge of the outline. Conversely if there is a tumor present, the barium shadow will contain a "hole."

Barium enema
A barium liquid is very effective up to the beginning of the large intestine. However, it is not very efficient at showing up the last section of the intestine. This is because the barium sulfate becomes mixed up with gastric juices by the time it gets there, with the result that it is no longer sufficiently concentrated. So in order to look at the large intestine, the doctor puts the barium sulfate into the

X ray of a barium meal (white area) in the intestine

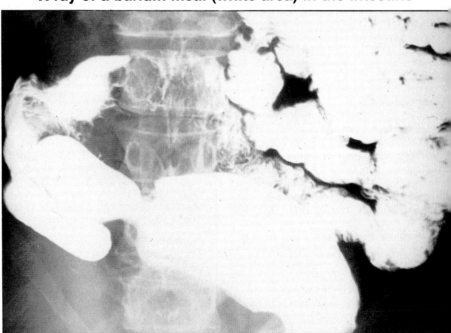

body by means of an enema into the anus, from where it travels to the large intestine. This barium enema is used to identify tumors, diverticulitis (see Diverticulitis), and other bowel disorders.

For best results the colon should be free of fecal material, so the patient may be kept on a restricted diet for two days before the examination and given a cleansing enema before the process begins. At the end of the investigation, another enema is given to remove most of the barium.

Barium swallow

If the problem is located in the throat or esophagus (the canal from mouth to stomach), a barium swallow may be given instead. This is similar to a barium meal, but is smaller, as the mixture does not have to travel so far. A barium swallow is used to identify a range of problems, including spasm of the esophagus, swallowing difficulties, and some tumors.

Timing

The exact timing of the barium meal and the taking of the X rays depends on which part of the alimentary canal (the route that food takes from mouth to anus) the doctor wants to examine.

Sometimes it is necessary for the patient to be X-rayed in several different positions. He or she may also be given a mixture to produce gas in the bowel and asked to roll from one side to the other, or even roll over, to make certain that the barium coats the whole lining of the bowel, with no gaps.

Examining the small intestine

For routine investigations of the small intestine, the X rays are timed to coincide with the normal time frame of digestion. Once the barium has passed through the stomach, X-ray pictures of the small intestine are taken at half-hour intervals for about three hours.

After the X rays

The barium liquid becomes firmer as water is drawn from it in the large intestine during the normal process of digestion. Depending on how much liquid is drawn out, it may become a hard, impacted mass that is difficult to pass as feces, and constipation (see Constipation) may develop. Patients are advised to drink plenty of liquids and eat fiber-rich food.

If necessary, a laxative may be prescribed. The feces may be covered in a white residue for a few days, but this is

Both the radiographer and the patient can follow the progress of the barium meal on the monitor. The X ray will be taken when the meal reaches the area causing concern.

nothing to worry about, and they will soon become normal again.

Once the X-ray film or photographs have been developed, the doctor will examine them in detail. He or she may then recommend further tests on any particular area of concern in the intestine. The patient will be informed and these tests arranged.

Possible problems

In a few cases some of the barium meal or swallow may "go down the wrong way"—it may travel into the patient's lungs rather than down the esophagus to the stomach—as sometimes happens when eating food. This will show on the X rays but is not a cause for concern, because the body will eliminate the barium from the lungs within 24 hours, and it will have no ill effects. Indeed barium used to be used in bronchograms (X rays of the lungs).

Barium may also escape through a perforation of the stomach into the abdomen. If the doctor suspects a perforation, he or she may decide to use gastrografin, an alternative to barium, instead, because this substance is considered to be even safer than barium if it escapes outside the alimentary canal.

What a barium meal, swallow, or enema can reveal

- pouches protruding from the lower part of the throat
- narrowing of the esophagus
- hiatus hernia
- ulcers of the stomach or duodenum
- bowel tumors or polyps
- diverticulitis
- Crohn's disease
- celiac disease
- ulcerative colitis

The future

While barium meals are still useful in diagnosing some conditions, they now tend to be replaced by methods that look directly at both ends of the intestinal tract. This is often done with fiber-optic endoscopy, where an optical viewing instrument is inserted into a natural orifice of the body, such as the throat or anus. This procedure has the advantage that a biopsy (the taking of a small sample of tissue for further examination) can be carried out at the same time.

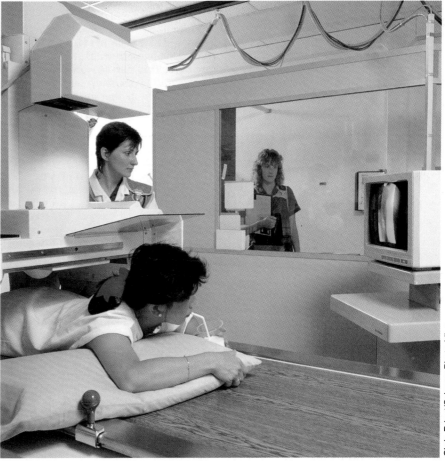

Chris Priest/Science Photo Library

Bedbugs

Q How can I make sure I don't get bedbugs in my home?

A Since bedbugs are usually spread through furniture, carefully examine any secondhand furniture you buy. If there are any telltale traces of eggs or clusters of insects in any cracks in the furniture, don't buy it. Keep your home in good repair so there are no cracks in the walls, where the bugs may live.

Q Why are bedbugs now said to be on the rise?

A Modern buildings are partly to blame. Plaster on walls did much to deter bedbugs, but now many buildings are built using prefabricated methods, which may provide little gaps between plasterboard, where bugs can hide.

Q How should I treat the bites from bedbugs?

A Soothing liquids like calamine lotion can help. If you think you have been bitten, it is sensible to visit your doctor so that he or she can examine the spots and give any necessary advice.

Q Can bedbugs travel from home to home?

A Only if the homes are attached (e.g., if they are in apartment buildings). Bedbugs do not travel outdoors unless they are in furniture that is being moved.

Q Where are bedbugs most likely to be found?

A Bedbugs are most likely to be found in places where secondhand furniture has been introduced without careful cleansing.

Q I never had bedbugs before I moved. All my furniture is new, so the bugs must have been here when I moved in or spread from other apartments. I feel embarrassed about talking to my neighbors. What can I do?

A Call in your local exterminator. He or she will talk with tact to everyone in the building.

Bedbugs are often thought to be a thing of the past, but in fact, they are on the rise and can live as easily in a clean home as in a dirty one.

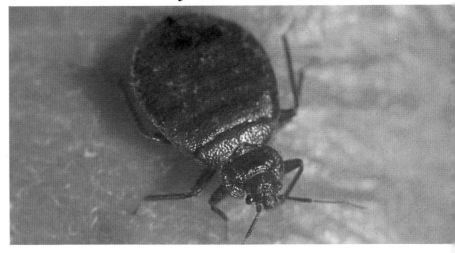

Bedbugs are brown creatures that feed at night on human blood. This magnified example is hungry, and when gorged, its flat body will become round and distended.

Bedbugs do not actually live in beds, but they do feed at night—and this is why you are likely to experience them in bed. They spend the day in cracks in walls, furniture, or behind wallpaper, where they are difficult to find. However, they can be seen with the naked eye, especially when they huddle together in clusters.

Identifying bedbugs

It is highly unlikely that your home is infested without you knowing it. But you may come across bedbugs without recognizing them for what they are.

Bedbugs are wingless, a rusty brown color, and approximately 3/16 in (5 mm) long. If a bedbug has not fed recently, it will be flat-shaped, but it swells up to become round after a meal of its chosen food—human blood—which it takes by biting a small hole in the skin, then sucking the blood out.

If your bedroom is infested, you will probably first notice a smear or two of blood on your bedding, then find you are suffering from bites. Although some people seem to be unaffected by the bedbug's bites, many find them extremely uncomfortable. They can result in swollen, itchy sores, which irritate so much that it is difficult to sleep.

Even if you are one of the lucky ones who do not react to bites, you will almost certainly be able to smell the bugs—they produce a strong and unpleasant odor.

Although the bites can be very uncomfortable, they are not dangerous and do not cause disease.

Living conditions

In the past bedbugs were associated with slum conditions, but it is now clear that they can live in the cleanest of homes, as long as there is some nook or cranny into which they can retreat during the day. They are hardy creatures with considerable survival power. In a cold, empty house, they can survive for more than a year without food by going into a kind of hibernation. They can even live for several months at freezing point.

The female lays her eggs in the cracks of walls or furniture at the rate of about three a day, and if well-fed, will produce up to 100 eggs in all. These hatch after three weeks, and the creatures reach the adult stage about 12 weeks after that.

Getting rid of bedbugs

Moving out of a room infested by bedbugs is unlikely to solve the problem. Nor will moving house, because they will almost certainly be lodging in the furniture you take with you. Killing them one by one is hopeless—too many get away.

The only answer is to contact a professional exterminator, either through the public health office or a commercial company. He or she will apply a powerful insecticide that will kill all the bugs immediately. Some bedbugs have developed a resistance to certain chemicals, so it is important to bring in an expert exterminator with access to a full range of appropriate insecticides.

Bedsores

Q My grandmother has been in bed for several weeks with rheumatism and is finding moving painful. She thinks she's getting a bedsore. Should she tell the doctor?

A Yes, definitely. If a bedsore is allowed to go untreated and the skin is broken, gangrene (where the body tissue dies and becomes putrid) can set in within a few hours.

Q If a patient is bedridden, should he or she be massaged to prevent bedsores?

A Massaging the patient is not as important as actually removing the weight from the pressure areas so that the blood supply can return. A patient who is unable to move should be turned every one or two hours, and a little light massage should be given to the area he or she has been lying on. This improves the circulation.

Q Can bedbug bites cause bedsores?

A Bedbugs will only cause sores if they bite at pressure points, like heels, shoulder blades, or the base of the spine, and this is unusual. But if they do, and the itchy bites are scratched, this may ulcerate the skin.

Q My elderly invalid grandfather has bedsores, which my mother frequently dresses. Will she catch them?

A No. Initially a bedsore is sterile, but once the skin is broken, a surface infection will start. This is caused by the germs that are naturally around on healthy skin, and they are not infectious.

Q I broke both my legs in a traffic accident and have to stay in bed. Am I too young at 17 to get bedsores?

A No. Anyone who is unable to move or who loses the sensation of pain is likely to develop bedsores. In young people this is rare, except as a result of broken bones or cut nerves.

Bedsores are caused by lying still in bed. They can affect anyone who is ill and who is therefore unable to move for some time. Prevention is better than cure—and only involves turning the patient every few hours.

One of the risks of bed rest is bedsores, otherwise called pressure sores. Pressure sores will develop on an invalid confined to a bed at the points where the body is in contact with the bed.

Although the whole body is lying on the mattress, its weight is not supported evenly. The weight falls on five main pressure points: the two heels, the bottom of the spine (the sacrum), and the two shoulder blades. Because they are bearing all the weight, the pressure becomes very high at these points, and once it is higher than the pressure forcing blood into that area, the blood vessels collapse, and the blood supply is cut off altogether.

Causes
With a healthy person, the sensation of pain caused by pressure at these points will make them turn over or move, even when asleep. But someone who has lost all sense of feeling will not receive any warning signals. This is likely to be the case, for example, with a patient who has had a stroke or a spinal cord injury.

Bedsores also affect the elderly, who feel the pain but are unable to move sufficiently to do anything about it. Often they are undernourished and lack the vitamins the body needs for healing.

Elderly people may have very little fat between the skin and bony points, which increases the pressure on those points. They also may be anemic (see Anemia), which means that the already-restricted blood supply is carrying less oxygen than

The shoulder blades, heels, and base of the spine are the pressure areas that are most likely to develop bedsores.

it would in a younger person. All of these factors make the problem worse and prevent quick healing.

Symptoms and dangers
If the patient is able to feel pain, he or she will experience soreness at the pressure point, and the skin will look red. If the patient is not moved, the redness darkens and gangrene follows. There is usually no bleeding, since the whole problem was caused in the first place by lack of blood supply. Poison will be produced, which gets absorbed into the body. Edema (swelling caused by retained fluid) is a further problem caused by big bedsores.

Prevention and treatment
Prevention is vital. Even the most severely ill can usually spend a couple of hours a day out of bed, sitting in a chair. This relieves all five pressure areas. Those who cannot move must be turned every one or two hours. Specialized equipment includes air mattresses with sections that can be alternately inflated and deflated to change the pressure-bearing areas while the patient lies still. Special sheepskins, rubber rings, and bed cradles can help.

Outlook
Once treated by dressing and antibiotics, even an acute bedsore will heal quickly on the young. A skin graft may also be used to speed the process. The elderly may not be so lucky. They need careful nursing to make the condition bearable.

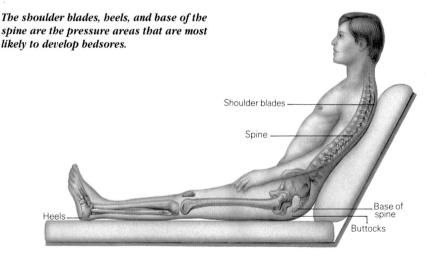

Shoulder blades

Spine

Heels

Base of spine

Buttocks

Mike Courteney

Behavior therapy

Q Can behavior therapy be used to cure alcoholism?

A Aversion therapy techniques, where the patient is trained to reject his or her habit by being made to associate it with something unpleasant, have been used for this purpose, and they can often achieve a temporary change of behavior. For instance, he or she may be given an electric shock every time a drink is poured. The improvement seldom lasts, however, because alcoholism is a physical addiction rather than a mental one, for which behavior therapy is unsuitable. Relapse into alcoholism after a cure is still the subject of much research and the problem has not yet been solved.

Q I have heard that hypnosis can be used with behavior therapy. Is this true?

A Hypnotism can be used when helping a patient to overcome irrational fears. Generally, however, hypnotism is not necessary; other relaxation methods used are usually sufficient.

Q If behavior therapy never looks for the cause of a problem, doesn't the removal of one symptom merely produce another one that expresses the conflict in a different way?

A Behaviorists believe that the symptom is the problem, and that there is no hidden conflict behind it, so other symptoms can't be produced unless they were there already. In practice, with the type of problems that behavior therapy treats effectively, alternative symptoms rarely appear. With other sorts of disturbance, however, the situation might well be different.

Q Is behavior therapy still widely used?

A Yes, largely because it has a good record of success, and it can easily be administered by a trained therapist. Behavior therapy shows results quickly if it is going to work at all, so it is always worth trying first for a suitable problem.

Behavior therapy is a type of treatment for people with various types of mental disturbance. Its methods are sometimes considered controversial, but in certain cases they do appear to work.

Behavior therapy is basically a common-sense approach to psychiatric problems. It takes little note of dreams, childhood experiences, or inner conflicts. Instead it concentrates on one method of cure: changing the patient's behavior through a technique called conditioning.

This approach is based on the belief that there is no more to a psychological problem than the symptoms it shows—an idea quite different from established psychotherapy, which says that to deal with any mental disorder, the cause must be discovered before the problem can begin to be resolved.

Learning and unlearning

Central to the behaviorists' ideas is the belief that nearly every psychological disorder is simply a group of habits. Because these habits have all been learned at one time or another, they can also be unlearned. There is therefore no need to go back and find the original cause of the "wrong" behavior. Rather the patient can go straight into the actual therapy.

Simple techniques

Behavior therapy techniques are used on anxiety-caused behavior like phobias (irrational fears) and compulsions (strong urges), as well as on some sexual problems, stuttering, tics, and a range of other similar disorders.

The various processes that are used to change behavior are actually very simple. Most parents find that they have been

If behavior therapy is to be used to cure excessive anxiety, the therapist will train the patient in the art of relaxation and then work through increasingly scary fantasies.

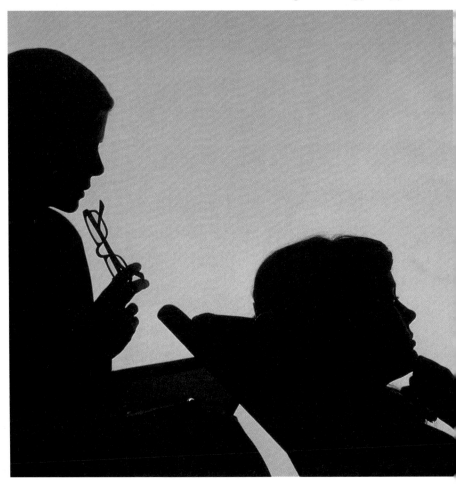

applying many of them automatically as they bring up their children.

The technique called aversion therapy is perhaps the most notorious, largely because of misconceptions about how it is carried out. Aversion therapy is used to treat antisocial behavior. It consists of pairing the compulsive situation—in other words, the trigger for the antisocial behavior—with some other experience that is unpleasant, such as a mild electric shock to the finger or foot or a nauseous feeling induced by an emetic.

After a number of repetitions, the previously exciting object or situation becomes associated in the patient's mind with the unpleasant feeling, thereby losing its former power.

Power of the imagination

Another similar form of therapy is carried out only in the patient's imagination. Called covert sensitization, it involves first asking the patient to imagine his or her excitement over the compulsive situation. He or she is then asked to follow this with images of being apprehended by the police, of the secret being discovered and talked about by family or friends, and other potentially humiliating and shameful situations.

When these scenes are at their most vivid, the therapist again presents the compulsive situation. After several repetitions, the two are firmly associated in the patient's mind, and the compulsive drive is gone forever.

Facing up to fears

The same system can also be worked the other way around, so that a particu-

Group therapy can help a person who is frightened of human contact to relax and lose her fear. She can gain confidence from being lifted by people she trusts.

larly pleasant situation is paired with something that has caused excessive anxiety. This process is called systematic desensitization.

A person who is terrified of spiders, for example, is first given training in how to relax deeply. With the help of the therapist, he or she learns to maintain this relaxed feeling through a series of increasingly scary fantasies involving spiders. After a few sessions, even the thought of a giant hairy spider crawling up their arm has no effect.

Reward and punishment

The idea of punishing bad behavior and rewarding good behavior has always been used in human society. At times the consistent application of reward and punishment—or operant conditioning, as it is called—can be most useful. The system works best, however, within a hospital or other confined place such as a prison, where it can be consistently applied and adequately controlled.

Token rewards

The same applies to the token economy system used in some psychiatric institutions, in which small tokens are issued to patients in return for useful behavior within the hospital community. These tokens can be exchanged later for candy, cigarettes, or the right to watch television, for example.

In addition to these forms of therapy, there are a number of other techniques used in behavior therapy, all of which work along similar lines. The most suitable technique is chosen in each case.

Suitable cases for treatment

These techniques do not claim 100 percent success, but they do have an impressive cure rate. Behavior therapy is at its best when there are specific neurotic symptoms to be changed. It is less

successful with psychoses (such as general emotional or mental disorder or chronic mood disruption), psychopathic behavior, or personality disintegration (schizophrenia). But even with these conditions, some aspects of the behavior may be successfully changed.

Chances of success

Not every patient benefits equally from behavior therapy, even when the circumstances are most favorable. This is probably because people vary in their response to conditioning. And behavior therapy is powerful conditioning.

Also, this therapy is a learning system that is fighting against years of "wrong" conditioning. It is asking a lot that a few weeks of therapy should prevail against such pressure. It is essential that after treatment has finished, the conditions the patient meets in the outside world reinforce the new behavior.

Is it brainwashing?

Behavior therapy is sometimes criticized on the grounds that it is inhumane and manipulative and could even result in political manipulation of society. Indeed by conditioning people into new behavior through the use of reward and punishment, behavior therapy does bear a similarity to brainwashing. But there are some very important differences, primary among which is that the patient usually wants to change his or her behavior and cooperates fully with the treatment.

Voluntary patients

Most behavior therapy takes place under voluntary circumstances. Before treatment starts, the particular technique is explained to the patient, and in effect a contract is drawn up setting out what the therapist will do. The patient's cooperation during treatment is always sought, and he or she can stop coming for treatment at any time. In other words nothing is done without the patient's consent, and he or she remains in control of the treatment at all times.

Hospital treatment

The situation within a hospital is different, because the patient is in a community with its own rules, and his or her mental condition may be such that he or she may not be able to cooperate. In such cases, the consent of the patient's relatives is sought, and the treatment, including possible alternatives, is discussed in detail with them. If relatives are not available, the decision on a course of treatment is taken not just by one doctor but several, and is carefully monitored as it progresses to insure that the patient is benefiting and making progress.

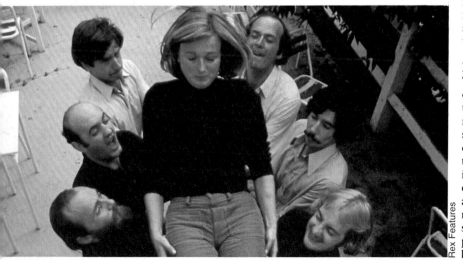

Rex Features

Bends

Q I have just started scuba diving. Am I likely to suffer from the bends?

A If you do not dive deeper than 30 ft (9 m), the problem of the bends does not arise. The risk increases the deeper you dive, the longer you stay down, and the number of times you dive. But the danger of the bends is easily avoided by surfacing slowly. You should only learn to dive under expert supervision. Providing you follow the correct procedure, diving need not be dangerous.

Q My brother wants to get a job as a deep-sea diver, working from an offshore oil rig. Isn't this a hazardous job because of the bends?

A Commercial diving techniques have undergone great improvements in recent years, and there is strict attention to safety. Deep-sea diving is a hazardous job but no more so than many others, and undersea exploration in different forms produces many job opportunities for divers.

Q Is getting the bends the only danger for a diver?

A No, there are other hazards. Among these are heat loss, mental stress caused by rapid compression, and lung damage. However, medical and safety checks normally enable the diver to avoid all these problems.

Q I am interested in learning to dive. Do I need to join a diving club or can I just get some tips from friends who have been diving for some time?

A It is essential that diving is done under expert supervision. If you are diving deeper than 30 ft (9 m), you must follow a strict timetable that takes into account the depth you are diving, how long you have stayed down, and how many times you have dived that day. Decompression times must be worked out accurately so that you can avoid all danger of the bends.

If a diver comes from deep water to the surface too quickly, he or she is likely to suffer from decompression sickness, commonly called "the bends."

One of the biggest problems facing a deep-sea diver is the enormous pressure of the sea itself, and the deeper he or she goes down, the greater this weight of water becomes.

In order to continue to get sufficient oxygen into the lungs, a diver breathes gases that have been bottled at pressure. This keeps the lungs at the same pressure as the surrounding water.

The pressure of the oxygen, nitrogen, and other gases causes larger than usual amounts to be dissolved in the bloodstream. This is in itself harmless, as long as the diver remains at a given depth. The problems begin when he or she has to come to the surface, with the accompanying reduction in pressure.

Bubble formation

If the diver surfaces too quickly for some reason, the sudden drop in pressure causes the gases—especially nitrogen—that have been dissolved in the blood to expand rapidly. The lungs cannot exhale these gases fast enough, so they form into bubbles in the bloodstream. The bubbles tend to interrupt the blood flow, causing terrible pain. And because the resulting pain from the bubbles in the knee, shoulder, and elbow joints is eased by bending over, the condition is often called "the bends." Its proper medical name is *decompression sickness*, and it can also affect aviators who have to make rapid ascents in flight.

Further effects

Bubbles, with pockets of clotted blood forming around them, can block arteries or reach the heart. If they form at crucial points in the nervous system, they can cause permanent paralysis. Even in a mild form, these bubbles can be very painful, leading to skin rashes and irritation, breathing difficulties, and nausea.

Avoiding the bends

The answer to the problem is to avoid rapid decompression. The body can then dispose of the excess gases through the lungs at its own rate.

Industrial diving

Industrial divers, working at great depths on offshore oil rigs, often remain submerged in diving bells (capsules) for more than 10 hours. After each shift they return to a large, pressurized container

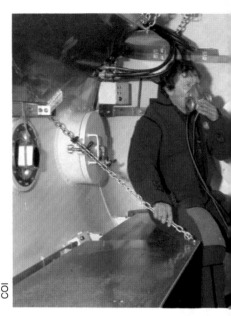

Industrial divers need to rest in a decompression chamber, inhaling oxygen for a time after their work is finished.

on the deck of their support ship or oil rig. There, still at pressure, they can eat and rest, while the pressure is gradually and safely reduced to normal.

Up to a depth of 30 ft (9 m), a diver can return to the surface at any speed without the need for decompression. At greater depths, the diver's body absorbs more and more compressed breathing mixture. So the deeper he or she goes and the longer the time spent submerged, the longer the decompression time.

Sports diving

People who dive for fun are unlikely to meet such problems. They will only be going down to limited depths for brief dives. Any danger of bends can be avoided by pausing at intervals during the return to the surface. If in any doubt, they can allow their bodies to decompress according to a strict timetable (available from diving clubs) that can be carried on a card strapped to the wrist.

If a diver fails to decompress correctly, he or she can be cured by returning to pressure—this means being put in a pressure chamber—then, under medical supervision, decompressing at a steady rate. But as may be imagined, this is an unwieldy process, and prevention is always better than the cure.

Bile

Q My father has to go into the hospital soon to have his gallbladder removed. Will he be able to eat normally afterward?

A The digestive system can manage remarkably well without a gallbladder. Normally bile made in the liver is stored in the gallbladder before being sent to the duodenum to help with the digestion of fats. When the gallbladder has been removed, the bile simply passes straight into the duodenum. This bile is less concentrated than normal, which means that it may be less efficient in its job, so the doctor will probably advise him to go easy on fatty foods and to eat smaller, but more frequent, meals to begin with. In a very short time, he will probably find that his body becomes totally readjusted to the new circumstances, and he will be able to eat normally.

Q Are there really two different kinds of bile?

A This is a hangover from the early days of medicine. The ancient Greeks believed that bile could be black or yellow. Too much black bile was supposed to cause depression, while too much yellow bile made a person irritable. We now know that there is only one sort of bile, which is greenish yellow in color. The word *bilious*, however, still has its meaning of peevish or bad-tempered.

Q Does feeling bilious indicate a bile problem?

A In a bilious attack what often happens is that the duodenum, the first part of the small intestine into which bile is released from the gallbladder, becomes irritated and distended by infection—or by too much food and drink. The bitter, bile-containing fluid in the duodenum gets flushed back into the stomach, resulting in nausea and vomiting. The bitter taste in the mouth and the greenish color of the vomit are due to the presence of bile. So a bilious attack means bile is in the wrong place, not that there is something wrong with its production.

This bitter-tasting substance is manufactured by the liver and stored in the gallbladder. It plays a very important role in the digestive process, and its importance has been recognized since the early days of medicine.

Bile is a thick, bitter, greenish yellow fluid that is made in the liver and stored in the gallbladder. Released from the gallbladder into the small intestine in response to the presence of food, it is essential to the digestion of fats. Bile also contains the remnants of worn-out blood cells and is, therefore, also part of the body's excretory, or waste-disposal, system. Everyday, the liver produces about 2.1 pints (1 liter) of

Without bile the body could not digest fats. Bile is made in the liver, stored in the gallbladder, and works in the intestine. Bile salts return to the liver in the blood of the portal vein twice during digestion.

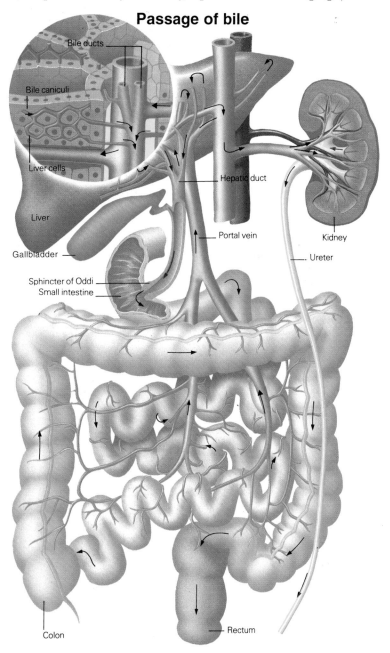

Passage of bile

Bile ducts

Bile caniculi

Liver cells

Liver

Gallbladder

Sphincter of Oddi

Small intestine

Hepatic duct

Portal vein

Kidney

Ureter

Colon

Rectum

Venner Artists

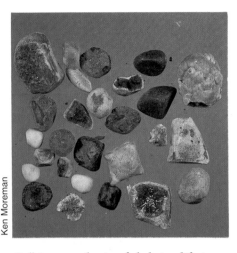

Ken Moreman

Gallstones are lumps of cholesterol that form in the gallbladder and may make its removal necessary.

bile. Although it consists of over 95 percent water, bile contains a great variety of chemicals, including bile salts, mineral salts, cholesterol, and the bile pigments that give the bile its characteristic greenish yellow color.

Bile is made continuously, in small quantities, by every cell in the liver. As it flows from the cells, it collects between groups of liver cells in minute channels called bile caniculi. These channels empty into bile ducts, or tubes, placed between the lobes, or projecting parts, of the liver. From the bile ducts, bile drains into exit tubes called the hepatic ducts. Unless bile is needed immediately for

Bile is a greenish fluid, simulated here to show how its emulsifying salts act like detergents. They physically break down globules of fat during digestion.

digestion, it flows into the gallbladder, a storage sac located under the liver.

Bile and digestion

The bile remains in the gallbladder until it is time for it to play its part in the digestive process. As food—particularly fatty food—enters the duodenum (the first portion of the intestine) from the stomach, the duodenum (see Duodenum) makes a hormone called cholecystokinin.

This hormone travels in the bloodstream to the gallbladder and makes its walls contract so that bile is squeezed out. The bile then flows down another tube, the common bile duct, and through a narrow gap, the sphincter of Oddi, which lets bile into the small intestine.

Bile's mineral salts, which include bicarbonate, then neutralize the acidity of partly digested food in the stomach. The bile salts, chemicals called sodium glycocholate and sodium taurocholate, break down fats so that the digestive chemicals (enzymes) can do their work.

Ferrying action

In addition to this detergentlike action, the bile salts are also believed to act as "ferries" further down the intestine, enabling digested fats to travel through the intestinal wall. They are also carriers of the vitamins A, D, E, and K.

The body is very conservative in its use of bile salts. They are not destroyed after use; instead 80 to 90 percent of them are carried back to the liver in the blood, where they stimulate the secretion of more bile and are used again.

Many colors

Bile gets its color from the presence of a pigment called bilirubin. One of the

many jobs of the liver is to break down worn-out red blood cells. As this happens, the red pigment hemoglobin in the cells is chemically split and forms the green pigment biliverdin, which is quickly converted to the yellow-brown bilirubin.

The greenish tinge of bile comes from unconverted biliverdin. In addition to pigmenting the bile, bilirubin colors and partially deodorizes the feces and also encourages the intestine to work as effectively as possible.

Bile pigment is also partly responsible for the yellow color of urine. In the intestine, bilirubin is attacked by bacteria (minute living creatures) permanently stationed there and converted to a chemical known as uribilinogen, which is carried to the kidneys before being released in the urine.

Problems in bile production

When something is wrong with the liver or gallbladder, bilirubin tends to accumulate in the blood and the skin, and the whites of the eyes look yellow. Because too little bile is reaching the intestines, the feces may be a pale, grayish color.

Gallstones

Even if the liver's bile production system is working normally, things can go wrong in the gallbladder. Most notorious of gallbladder problems are gallstones. These hard lumps of a chemical substance called cholesterol form in the gallbladder and may travel down the bile duct into the duodenum. The gallbladder becomes inflamed and the movement of the stones down the bile duct can be very painful.

Treatment

The treatment of the different bile problems and related diseases depends on their cause. Liver infections and cirrhosis (see Cirrhosis) of the liver are difficult to treat with drugs, and the usual cure is rest, no alcohol, and a nourishing diet.

Surgery is sometimes the only way of treating gallbladder problems, and in the case of gallstones, this means removing not just the stones but the whole gallbladder. Unless the gallstones are so severe that they are a medical emergency, the doctor may first advise a low-fat diet to reduce stress on the digestive system and lower the amount of cholesterol in the blood.

When surgery is the only permanent answer to gallbladder problems, the body is able to manage without this piece of digestive apparatus. Sufferers from chronic gallstones find remarkable relief from their previous symptoms of pain and discomfort. With the disappearance of the gallbladder, the body's tendency to make stones of cholesterol vanishes.

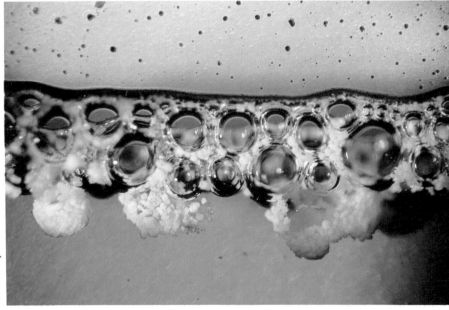

Paul Brierley

Biofeedback

Q I have trouble falling asleep a lot of the time. Would biofeedback be better for my insomnia than sleeping pills?

A Yes, it is certainly worth trying. Because biofeedback has no side effects and is nonhabit-forming, it has the advantage over many of the sedative-type drugs that are prescribed for sleeplessness. Ask your doctor to recommend one of the newer, handheld biofeedback monitors.

Q My father has high blood pressure and almost died from it when he was younger. He has been treated with drugs for most of his life and is now 59. Is it too late for him to try biofeedback?

A It is not too late to try a therapy that may improve your father's condition and reduce his dependency on prescription drugs, as long as he is fit enough to be a conscious participant in the treatment. Biofeedback has been very successful in the control of high blood pressure, or hypertension, in many cases. But it is extremely important that he consults his doctor before undertaking any new treatment, which should always be carried out under medical supervision. Hypertension is too serious a condition for your father to treat by himself.

Q I seriously stretched a tendon playing basketball and have had to stop playing. I've heard that biofeedback can somehow help sports injuries. Is this true?

A It may be useful for you to try. Biofeedback is mainly used in the prevention of symptoms caused by tension, but if you are in a lot of pain and worried about it, you may find some relief by trying relaxation techniques, together with biofeedback. A biofeedback monitor called an electromyograph (or EMG) measures muscle contractions via electrodes placed on the skin; the resulting feedback may enable you to learn to control muscle spasms.

By using biofeedback techniques, it is possible to learn to control the physiological and mental functions of the autonomic nervous system to help combat a variety of medical conditions, including high blood pressure.

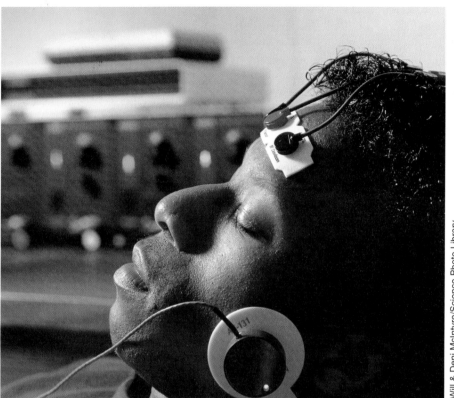

Will & Deni McIntyre/Science Photo Library

This man is undergoing biofeedback therapy. His physiological responses, such as his pulse rate, are being monitored via electrodes attached to his head.

Biofeedback is a type of therapy whereby information about an individual's physiological processes is monitored to make a person aware of functions that he or she is not normally conscious of. These functions consist mainly of those of the autonomic nervous system and include heart rate and blood pressure (cardiovascular activity), temperature, brain waves, breathing, and muscle tension.

Special equipment is used to monitor these physiological activities, and then the information is fed back to the person so that he or she can learn to control the symptoms of a number of illnesses, most of which are stress related. Psychotherapy is often used in conjunction with biofeedback in order to help a patient understand why he or she is stressed and how his or her body reacts to stress in certain ways.

Biofeedback monitoring and therapy have been shown to be especially useful in relieving the symptoms of hypertension (high blood pressure),

migraine headaches, insomnia, hyperventilation (rapid, excessive breathing, often leading to blackout), anxiety due to stress, and some kinds of joint and muscle pain. In addition it has been used in the treatment of epilepsy.

Stress and anxiety

Stress is a fact of life that affects everyone to some degree. There are many situations, people, and events that a person may feel threatened by, and these stresses lead to certain physical changes. A person's response to what he or she may perceive as a threat can trigger an increase in heart rate, dilation of the blood vessels that supply the skeletal muscles, dilation of the bronchi in the lungs, slowing of the digestion, and an increase in sweat and pupil dilation.

Q I have a very demanding job and lately I have been having panic attacks. This is very embarrassing and doesn't do my professional reputation any good. Can biofeedback help in any way?

A Yes, biofeedback can help with panic attacks and with the control of hyperventilation (heavy, rapid breathing that can lead to dizziness or fainting) that sometimes occurs with them. Handheld monitors can help you measure how fast your heart is beating so that you can learn to recognize the signs of a panic attack and slow your heartbeat and therefore your breathing, before a full attack hits you. Relaxation techniques, especially deep breathing, should be used in conjunction with biofeedback.

Q My brother wants to try biofeedback before he takes his college exams. He says it will boost his memory. Is there any truth to this?

A Some biofeedback experiments have shown that if a person can learn to consciously go into the alpha state, that is, a relaxed, meditative state similar to the one experienced while falling asleep, it is possible for him or her to think more clearly, remain calmer, and therefore function more efficiently overall. In addition a technique associated with biofeedback called theta wave training has been used to overcome the mental blocks experienced during exams. If your brother practices these techniques both before he studies, and then again before his exams, he is likely to benefit from a reduction of pre-exam nerves, and can face them in a relaxed state of mind.

Q Is biofeedback one of those "quack" cures?

A It is not yet understood exactly why biofeedback works, but this does not make it a "quack" cure. Although it is a relatively new therapy, biofeedback has been proven effective in the treatment of many ailments, including migraines, hypertension, and insomnia.

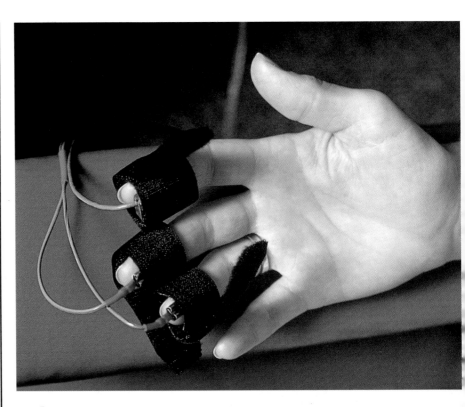

Patients with poor circulation or Raynaud's syndrome, where the extremities become numb, can learn to use biofeedback to raise their body temperature.

These changes in the body are sometimes called the "fight-or-flight" syndrome, a remnant of the days when humans were at risk from wild animals and literally had to fight for their lives. Today most people are not in much danger of being torn to pieces by a tiger, but the human response to danger signals is the same. The energy that builds up in preparation for a life-or-death fight remains unused, and the modern human being begins to "burn out" with stress; illness follows.

This is why relaxation is so important in the prevention of illness or in keeping existing conditions at bay. Biofeedback, practiced with relaxation techniques, can help with all stress-related problems.

How it works

A number of different monitoring devices may be used in biofeedback, depending on the condition being treated. But the basic way in which they work is the same: a physiological function such as the heart rate, brainwave activity, or muscle tension is monitored by the machine, and then the patient is made aware of the information clocked by that piece of equipment. The device may signal changing levels to the patient via a flashing light, a fluctuating needle, an aural tone, or music. Some biofeedback monitors may show a digital display, and in computerized systems, an on-screen picture may change as the patient relaxes.

After a certain amount of experience with the biofeedback monitor, the patient gradually becomes aware of how he or she feels when the monitor's signal changes. Relaxation techniques, such as deep breathing, may also be used to help induce changes in the monitor's signal.

In the beginning stages of biofeedback monitoring, a doctor or therapist is present to supervise the technique. But the ultimate goal is for the patient to learn to recognize when conscious control is needed over his or her own heart rate, breathing rate, etc., and to put into practice learned techniques at will, without the use of special equipment. By practicing biofeedback techniques over a period of time, this is possible. The amount of time it takes for any given individual to learn sufficient control cannot be predicted—it is different in each case.

Biofeedback monitors

There are several different types of biofeedback monitors that may be appropriate for use with different medical conditions. A doctor will decide on the patient's specific requirements.

Blood pressure biofeedback uses a machine called a mercury sphygmomanometer. A procedure much like the taking of a normal blood pressure reading is used, but the resulting blood flow is "listened to" by a tracking device, which then monitors the blood pressure, beat by beat. This signal is then translated into a sound, where the pitch varies with the changing blood pressure.

Another type of monitor reads electrical skin resistance, or ESR. Nervous tension can increase the amount a person perspires (as in the "sweaty-palm" syndrome), and when sensors are attached to the fingers or palms and then connected to an ESR monitoring device, the minute changes in sweat production can be translated to signal levels. ESR devices have also long been used by the police and large company employers as part of lie-detector tests.

Muscle tension can be measured using an instrument called an electromyograph, or EMG. Electrodes placed on the surface of the skin can measure electrical activity changes that take place during muscle contraction. But they may represent changes to more than one muscle or muscle group; thus, it may sometimes be

difficult to be more specific in the monitoring of this type of tension.

The biofeedback monitor that is used to read brain wave patterns is called an electroencephalograph, or EEG. This instrument uses readings from electrodes taped to the patient's forehead. It is often used to aid migraine sufferers and those who suffer from epilepsy, insomnia, and some types of anxiety.

Temperature feedback monitors, as the name implies, provide the patient with information on body temperature. This can be useful in conditions like poor circulation, which causes a person to feel cold all the time.

Finally there are the more sophisticated instruments such as the "mind mirror" (a type of electroencephalograph), which produces an image of what is going on in both hemispheres of the brain at the same time. This instrument can also be used to track and compare the activity in the same hemisphere of the brain in two different people at once.

Early research: autogenic training

Early studies showed that people could learn to raise or lower the temperature of their fingertips by using a technique called autogenic training. With this type of technique, the patient imagines that his or her finger is warmer or colder, and the accompanying physiological change should follow—the actual temperature of the finger should be raised or lowered. This could be accomplished without the use of equipment, but if monitors were used, it speeded the rate of progress.

A psychiatrist adjusts the settings on a computerized biofeedback monitor so that his patient may view visual feedback or hear auditory (sound) feedback.

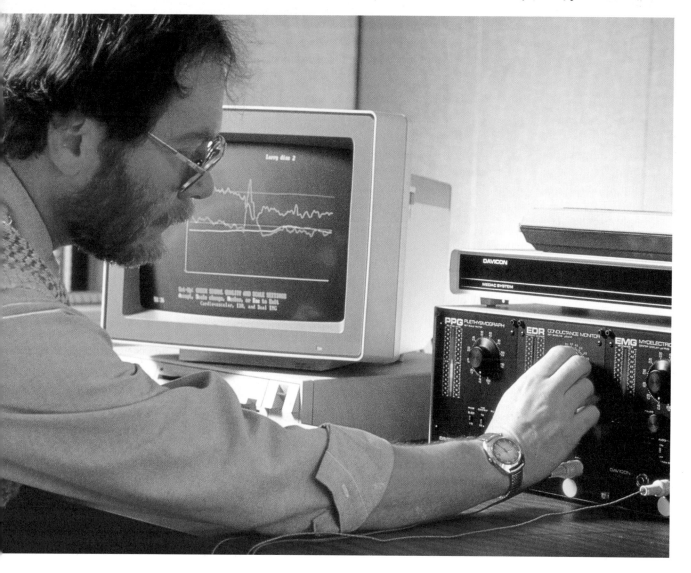

BIOFEEDBACK

Relaxation techniques are often used in conjunction with biofeedback. Focusing on one point, such as the glow from an electric lamp, can help a person relax.

Hypertension

Hypertension is a condition where a person's blood pressure is consistently higher than 140/90. One of the most common illnesses in the United States today, it affects more men than women and stems from many causes. If left untreated, hypertension can lead to strokes and heart attacks.

Drugs given to hypertensive patients usually include diuretics (see Diuretics), which reduce body fluid levels, together with vasodilators (drugs that increase the dilation of blood vessels), and beta-blockers, which get their name from their effect of blocking the action of adrenaline, thus slowing the blood pressure.

While drug therapy is effective and essential in many cases, the long-term, accumulative effects of its use can lead to problems in later life, especially with the kidneys. Biofeedback treatment can be used to control the condition and cut down on the amount of drugs a patient needs to take—in some cases it may be possible to cut out drugs altogether.

An initial assessment of the patient's condition will be made by a doctor or psychiatrist, and the decision will be made as to whether biofeedback is suitable for him or her. Where a patient's blood pressure must be monitored, the patient will be asked to sit on a chair, and a blood pressure cuff will be placed around his or her arm. The blood pressure will be taken and the rate of the heartbeat is then tracked; this produces a changing pitch on the monitor.

Through a process of trial and error, the patient will eventually learn to bring his or her blood pressure under voluntary control. When used together with relaxation training, the results will be even more successful. Even if the hypertension is due to physiological causes, lowering the overall stress levels is beneficial.

Migraine

An especially intense form of headache, a migraine is extremely painful, and the person suffering from it may be totally debilitated by an attack. Migraines can be caused by food, allergies, alcohol, the prolonged use of computer screens and other equipment that causes eyestrain, and the sun, but in many cases they are brought on by stress. Attacks frequently occur after a period of relaxation,

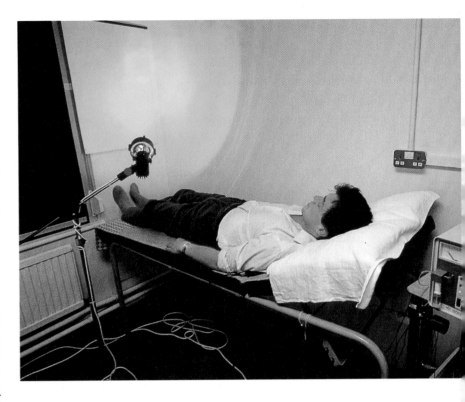

following a time of prolonged, acute physical or mental stress.

Symptoms of migraines (see Migraine) include a throbbing, blinding pain behind the eyes, nausea, and sensitivity to light (photosensitivity) and sound. Often the patient must lie in a darkened room until the symptoms subside.

Drugs such as ibuprofen can be effective but only if taken in the initial stages of the headache, because the stomach shuts down as the pain increases. But for those who are regular sufferers, prevention can be sought with biofeedback.

In the case of brain wave monitoring for conditions such as migraine, the patient is connected to an EEG (see Electroencephalogram). Small sensors are attached to his or her temples and information about the electrical activity in the brain is recorded, monitored, and fed back to the patient.

Other conditions

Some other medical conditions may benefit from relaxation techniques and biofeedback training. These include insomnia, nervous tics, and colitis (gastrointestinal cramping).

Epilepsy is a condition where the electrical activity in the brain becomes uncontrolled, and the sufferer may have periodic convulsive seizures, sensory disturbances, and loss of consciousness. Although it is not possible to cure the disorder with biofeedback techniques, the frequency and severity of the seizures can be brought partially under control,

and this is good news for those who suffer from epilepsy, because the seizures are often dangerous.

Raynaud's syndrome, which is brought on by cold or emotional stress, is a disease in which the extremities, especially the fingers, become numb; they may turn red and burn; or they may become white and eventually black. Normal sensation can be restored by heating the fingers, so a biofeedback technique that helps the patient to raise his or her body temperature at will can be very helpful in preventing full-blown attacks.

Outlook

Although it is not currently understood exactly how biofeedback works, literally thousands of scientific studies have shown that these techniques are an aid in the treatment of many tension related medical conditions and in the reduction of illness-inducing stress. Many patients suffering from high blood pressure have been able to wean themselves off medication, and migraine sufferers have learned to recognize the danger signs of an upcoming attack in order to keep it at bay.

Through continuing research in the field of psychoneuroimmunology—the science of how the mind, brain, and body connect and function together—the enigmatic workings of the autonomic nervous system are being rapidly unraveled, and fascinating advances are being made daily.

Biological clocks

Q Why is it that so many people seem to die during the early hours of the morning?

A Our biological clocks program us to be most relaxed at that time, and the senses that warn us of abnormal body states (cold, lack of oxygen, etc.) are at their least efficient. Yet, because the body is most relaxed and the ability to tolerate pain is high, this is also the time when most babies are born.

Q Sometimes I feel sleepy in the afternoon for no apparent reason. Why? Are there "day people" and "night people"?

A Provided you haven't eaten or drunk too much at lunchtime, your biological clock may be running fast or slow, and thus creating a sleep deficit, so your afternoon sleepiness may signal the body's need for extra rest. As for "day" and "night" people, it is known that there are "owls," who stay up late because their clock is running slow, and "larks," who wake up early because their clock is running fast.

Q Is it true that working on alternating late and early shifts is bad for people such as doctors in the long run?

A Shift work does cause troubles at first because every time the shift is changed, the biological clock has to be reset, and this can produce unexpected tiredness, restlessness, irritability, and stomach acidity. In the long run, however, effects are more variable. Some people find it impossible to adapt to continually changing cycles and are best staying with day work. Others seem to be able to adapt without too much difficulty.

Q No matter where I am or what I am doing, I get a craving to eat at 2:00 P.M. every day. Why is this?

A Your body clock has adjusted itself to make you feel hungry, because this is probably the time of day when you usually eat a meal. It is possible to change this over time.

Like plants and animals, we possess internal clocks that govern our eating, sleeping, and waking times. However, unlike plants and animals, we are able to reset them to fit in more usefully with everyday life.

Many people find that they wake up early on weekends even when they have the chance to sleep late. Others suffer from jet lag when they fly long distances. Some women get somewhat irritable at certain times of the month or find that their hair sometimes becomes oilier than usual. All may have one thing in common: they are feeling the effects of one or more of the so-called biological clocks within their bodies.

However, these clocks do not have to rule our lives. For example, it is possible to learn to "set" them in order to wake up at a certain time.

Primitive origins

The existence of rhythmic cycles in the behavior of animals and plants, as well as in humans, has, of course, been known for hundreds of years. Yet, in spite of their familiarity, we still know very little about how they work beyond the fact that they are probably genetically coded (that is, built-in as the result of instructions from the genes we acquire at the moment of conception), and that they act by releasing hormones into the body.

The effects

All humans show evidence of daily and monthly cycles in their behavior. The regularity of the sleep cycle is the most obvious example, but the oxygen intake rate, urine excretion rate, the amount of sugar in the blood, and the levels of adrenaline and many other chemicals, all vary over approximately 24 hours, as do both the

When are you best at multiplication?

On average, people are most accurate between 10:00 A.M. and noon. This level of accuracy falls gradually until midnight.

The cycle begins again, provided you have had a normal night's sleep, at 6:00 A.M.—the time of least accuracy.

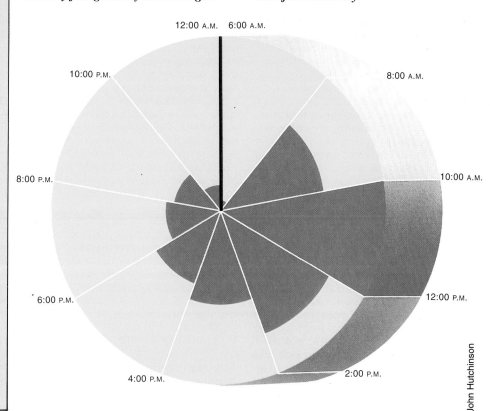

John Hutchinson

resting pulse rate and the temperature of the body.

Tolerance to pain is, perhaps unexpectedly, highest at about midnight. Alcohol is broken down by the body much more slowly between 2:00 A.M. and 2:00 P.M., and the effect is therefore felt much longer between these hours, which may partially explain why lunchtime drinking can affect working ability so noticeably.

The monthly biological clock is most clearly shown in a woman's menstrual cycle (see Menstruation). This cycle affects both the physical state—changes in weight, body-fluid retention, skin and hair condition—and the psychological state, so that moods of depression, sudden irritability, or nervousness may occur.

The evidence that these periodic changes are controlled by internal mechanisms, rather than by the cycles of darkness and light or changes in external temperature, is fairly strong, although it is known that humans are more able to adapt their biological clock messages to suit their environment than are animals and plants.

This is not to say that the environment has no effect on human biological clocks. At first, babies fall asleep and wake up with complete disregard for either the day/night cycle or their parents' behavior, but they establish a regular pattern of sleeping and waking that is more or less 24 hours long from about six weeks.

Two experiences that demand a drastic altering of the biological clock are doing shift work and flying to a country in a different time zone. A change in the activity/rest cycle is inevitable.

Fast and slow clocks

Since not everyone's daily cycle covers exactly 24 hours, it follows that many people will need to adjust their biological clocks regularly in order to synchronize with the external clock by which we all have to live. In extreme cases, an individual's daily clock may run fast or slow by as much as half an hour a day, which helps to account for some very common, if puzzling, minor difficulties in sustaining regular sleeping patterns.

If an individual's daily biological clock runs a little fast, that person will tend to become sleepy early in the evening but will be able to wake at a reasonable time in the morning with little difficulty. This type of individual is often known as a "lark." The normal exposure to the day/night cycle of the outside world will help him or her to reset the clock each day—humans can do this more easily than animals—otherwise he or she would end up going to bed earlier and earlier, and getting up earlier and earlier.

How blood pressure and temperature change through the day

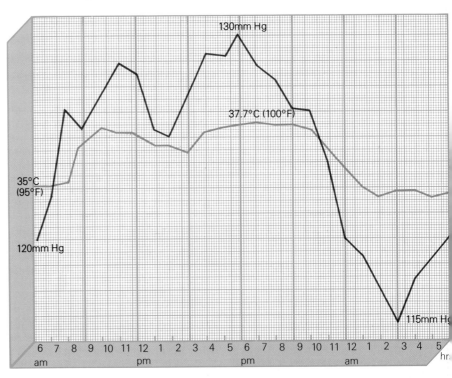

Because of this need to readjust the internal clock, however, the individual is continually under pressure from the external everyday environment. "Larks" therefore have to try to compensate for the sleep deficit that gradually builds up by taking an occasional afternoon nap or going to bed extra early from time to time. Studies have also shown that "early to bed, early to rise" people are generally shier, more reserved, and more anxious than "late to bed, late to rise" people.

An individual whose clock is running slow, on the other hand, has another sort of problem. He or she can stay up until the early hours without difficulty, because the internal clock signals bedtime later and later each night. However, he or she will find getting up in the morning far more of an ordeal than does the "lark." This group is often known as "owls." The built-up sleep deficit is generally useless, for in the evening there is no message from the biological clock signaling sleep, and he or she will therefore often lie awake in bed. Getting up a little later occasionally may be beneficial.

In both of these cases, if problems persist with sleep/wake cycles or with jet lag, the doctor can prescribe a drug to help to reset the biological clock.

The reasons for biological clocks

Animals are thought to have developed biological clocks because they help a species to survive. The clocks discourage activity during darkness, when their owners are more vulnerable to predators because of reduced vision. They also order the cycles of fertility to maximize breeding efficiency, and the clocks regularize migration or hibernation, and thus, offset the effect of adverse weather conditions or reduced food supplies on the animal to enhance its chance of survival.

Humans have retained the daily and monthly clock for what was probably much the same set of reasons; however, the clocks now help with our regular habits. For example, we eat at certain times, and with a signal from the biological clock, the body produces gastric juices at the right time in order to digest that food. At night, the clock reduces the speed at which urine accumulates in the bladder so that we are less likely to have our sleep disturbed by having to get up and go to the bathroom.

Exploiting the biological clock

Some people are able to wake up from normal sleep at any given time with remarkable punctuality, even when cues such as light, birdsong, or traffic noise have been eliminated. Experiments using hypnotic sleep show that, with practice, this accuracy can be increased and that indeed, the clock will alert the person to perform an action at a certain time. Even without external help, it is possible to develop this ability simply by being aware of it and practicing it.

Biopsy

A biopsy is a simple method of taking tissue from a lump or various parts of the body and testing it to see what, if anything, is wrong. This invaluable aid to diagnosis is instrumental in saving lives.

Q I contracted hepatitis while on vacation in the Far East. Why is my doctor sending me for liver biopsy when the cure is simply diet and rest?

A For most types of hepatitis (an inflammation of the liver), it is true that there is no treatment except diet and rest. However, a biopsy can diagnose different types of hepatitis, some of which can be treated in other ways.

Q I have to have a biopsy soon. Will it be painful?

A A biopsy through the skin is done under local anesthetic, so no pain is felt at the time. The area will, however, feel bruised when the anesthetic wears off a few hours later. A biopsy done with an internal viewing instrument is uncomfortable, but not painful.

Q I have a lump in my breast that my doctor thinks is not cancer. Why has she sent me to the hospital for a biopsy?

A Breast cancer starts as a small lump, so it is important to check such lumps for malignancy, no matter how benign they seem. The only sure way to do this is to biopsy the lump.

Q An X ray of my stomach apparently showed an ulcer. Now my doctor says it needs to be biopsied. How is this procedure done?

A The instrument used is a flexible tube containing a lighting and viewing system and a special remote-control forceps for doing the biopsy. The sedated patient swallows this, and the doctor can view the ulcer and cut off a small piece.

Q I had a biopsy taken of a mole on my leg and was told it was not malignant. How can I be sure this is true?

A Rest assured. The sample is put under a microscope and studied by a pathologist—a person trained in spotting the difference between benign and malignant cells.

With some diseases a comprehensive, detailed diagnosis is vital in order to insure that the treatment is entirely correct for the patient concerned. For example, there are many powerful drugs that can be used to treat cancer, and certain types of cancer respond better to one type of drug than to others. The only way to be sure which treatment is most appropriate is to biopsy the tumor.

A biopsy is typically carried out on a woman who finds a lump in one of her breasts. This could be either a breast cancer or a harmless cyst (see Cyst). The only way to be completely certain is to remove a bit of the lump and look at it under a microscope. A mammography (X ray of the breast) may be used as a less invasive form of tumor and cyst detection, but it is less accurate than a biopsy.

The technique

A biopsy may be performed through the skin or from the inside of the body using an instrument passed into the region where the problem is. Biopsies through the skin may be done as either "open" or "closed" operations.

An open operation means the skin is cut open and the surgeon parts the tissues to reach the lump or the organ to be biopsied. He or she then cuts out a small piece before stitching everything back together again.

A small lump just beneath the skin will be biopsied under local anesthetic. A lump occurring in a more difficult place, such as deep in the neck, will involve an operation with a general anesthetic.

In a closed operation, a special needle is pushed through the skin into the area to be biopsied. The needle cores out a tiny cylinder of tissue, which is drawn out along with the needle. It requires only a local anesthetic, and because the needle is small, no stitches are needed.

A biopsy from inside means the surgeon can see the organ or part of the body from which a piece of tissue is to be taken without having to perform an open

How a breast biopsy is carried out

Cutting edge of biopsy needle

Biopsy needle

Cyst

Nipple

Areola

In a breast biopsy, a local anesthetic is given and a sharp needle is used to penetrate the lump that is to be tested. A tiny section of tissue is then removed. A trained pathologist will then examine it under a powerful microscope in the laboratory.

Frank Kennard

159

operation. This is made possible by using a fiber-optic instrument—a flexible tube with a light and a telescopic lens at one end that transmits a picture along the tube's entire length when inserted into the body. The tube can slide between the body's organs, giving the doctor visual access to internal areas that previously had to be examined by opening the body.

It is therefore possible to look, via the mouth, at the start of the small intestine and at the organs in the abdomen and pelvis or, via the rectum, at the beginning of the large intestine. A fiber-optic instrument can also be used for viewing the lungs and can also carry a remote-controlled forceps for taking biopsy samples. As usual, only very tiny pieces are taken (usually less than one cubic millimeter), but several are needed to reduce any chance of error in the tests. The passage of this instrument into the body, although uncomfortable, is relatively pain-free, and the patient is given a tranquilizing drug before the operation.

Diagnosis

As soon as the tissue has been removed, it is taken to a pathology laboratory, where it is embedded in wax to preserve it. This is a long process, taking about 24 hours, and it insures that as much detail as possible is preserved.

The sample is then thinly sliced, stained a special color so it can be clearly seen, and mounted on a microscope slide. A general stain will show all the cells that make up the tissue, and special stains can be used to highlight differences between normal and abnormal cells. The pathologist can see if there are abnormal cells present and also what stage the disease (if there is one) has reached.

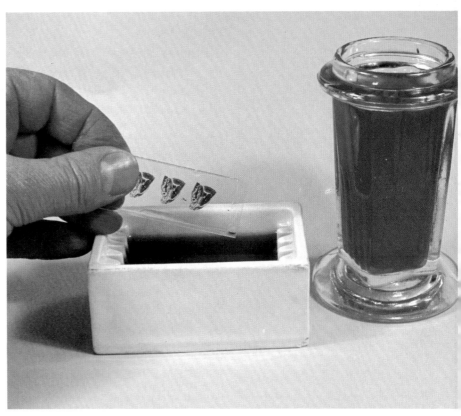

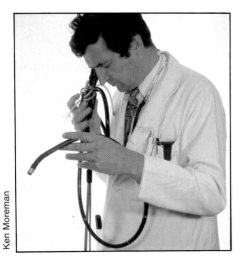

A fiber-optic endoscope is used to see into the stomach area. It can be fitted with a forceps to take tissue samples.

Ken Moreman

Freeze-fixing

If the biopsy has been taken at an open operation, the surgeon often needs to know exactly what the problem is before stitching up the wound. If, for example, a breast lump turns out to be cancerous, a further, larger operation is likely to be necessary. Rather than risk a second operation, it is obviously better to do everything at once, so the surgeon needs the biopsy result immediately.

Special freeze-fixing techniques have therefore been developed to process the tissue quickly, which makes a diagnosis possible within about 15 minutes. The answer is telephoned without delay from the pathology laboratory to the surgeon in the operating room, who can then proceed as necessary with the patient still under the general anesthetic. However, the quality of the microscope slides produced in this way is not as good as those produced by the usual method, so this system is not used for routine problems. A typical biopsy result takes about one week to obtain.

When is a biopsy necessary?

Biopsies are most often carried out on lumps in the body. It is sometimes difficult to be certain that a lump is benign (i.e., not malignant), so a biopsy is done. Biopsy of the liver or kidney is done when the organ is diseased and a more detailed diagnosis is needed before deciding on the appropriate treatment.

Staining is used to mark the various cells mounted on a microscope slide.

Where is a biopsy done?

Most biopsies are done in the hospital. A small lump under the skin can be biopsied in a matter of minutes in the outpatient department.

Open biopsies often involve a 24-hour stay in the hospital, but somtimes they are performed in the morning, and the patient can go home in the afternoon. Most internal biopsies using a fiber-optic instrument involve spending one day in the hospital. The procedure takes about half an hour, but the patient must remain in the hospital for a period of time after the biopsy is completed to allow for observation, and also until the effects of the tranquilizer have worn off. Organ biopsies are usually done as inpatient tests to allow for a longer period of observation in case of complications; there may also be other tests to be done on the patient at the same time as the biopsy.

Aftereffects

The aftereffects of a biopsy are virtually nonexistent, and so there is certainly nothing to worry about. The spot where the biopsy was taken may be a bit painful when the anesthetic wears off, but that usually lasts only a day or two. There may be some bleeding, which causes discoloration under the skin, but this usually disappears quite quickly.

Biorhythms

Biorhythms are said to underlie the patterns of human behavior. Understanding them can help people to plan their lives for optimum timing of important events.

Q Can biorhythms improve my relationship with my boyfriend?

A Yes, a knowledge of your own biorhythms and those of your boyfriend could certainly help your relationship run more smoothly. The most important biorhythm in all personal relationships is the emotional cycle, so compare yours with your boyfriend's. You could perhaps postpone meeting if this is going to coincide with a critical phase, and make allowances for each other in the negative phases.

Q I have an important exam coming up. Will my biorhythms affect my grade?

A Although you cannot alter the date of an exam, you can take some practical precautions to insure that you perform as well as possible, whatever the state of your biorhythms. Be sure to get a good night's sleep before the exam, and try to avoid any emotional upsets. Have everything ready in advance so that there is no last-minute panic. Of the three biorhythms, the intellectual cycle is the most important here. The more you exercise your mind, the better it will be able to resist the effects of the negative intellectual phase, should this coincide with your exam.

Q Can I do anything to change my biorhythms?

A No, you cannot alter the pattern of your biorhythms. The three cycles begin from the day you are born and continue in the same automatic rhythm throughout life. What you can do, however, is to be aware of where you are in your rhythms so that you can plan activities accordingly.

Q How can I tell the difference between my menstrual cycle and my emotional cycle?

A Your menstrual cycle is based on the dates of your periods, so you can keep track of these. Your emotional cycle begins from birth, and you can calculate this by dividing the number of days you have been alive by 28.

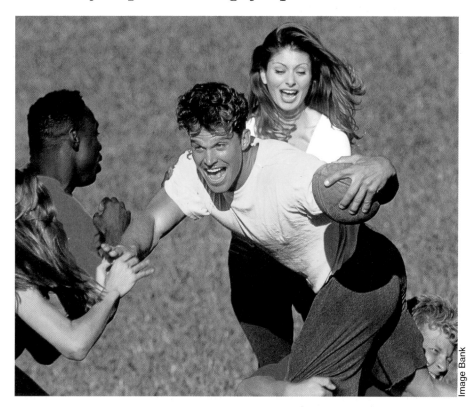

Most people have certain days when they feel good and perform well and other days when, for no apparent reason, they lack energy, cannot concentrate, and find themselves making mistakes that they would not normally make. Biorhythms are a way of explaining such variations in mood and behavior.

According to the biorhythm theory, human beings have three different cycles—physical, emotional, and intellectual—which rise and fall independently of each other. These three cycles work like three internal clocks, controlling people's physical well-being and behavior, their feelings, and their ability to think and reason.

The idea of cycles of growth and decline is, of course, nothing new. They are seen in nature in the four seasons, and also in a woman's menstrual cycle. Most people now accept that the menstrual cycle can have a great influence on a woman's behavior and physical and emotional states, which vary depending on where she is in the cycle.

If she is in the first half, a woman will often feel physically well, cheerful, and energetic. If she is in the latter half,

At times when the physical cycle is at its peak, optimum performance in sports and other activities that require physical energy can be achieved.

particularly the few days before the onset of her menstrual period, she may seem like a different person; she may be depressed and irritable, weepy, and accident-prone, among other symptoms.

There are also daily cycles that vary from one individual to another. Some people feel most dynamic and productive during the daytime hours, while others do not reach their peak until late at night. However, a few general rules have been observed. According to recent scientific research on human behavior patterns, it seems that the best time for most people to make decisions is around the middle of the day, and the best time to study or rehearse is just before going to bed.

It takes three to four weeks to complete all three biorhythmic cycles. By calculating the timing of the future highs and lows in each cycle, a person can predict how they are likely to feel and behave on any one day.

Image Bank

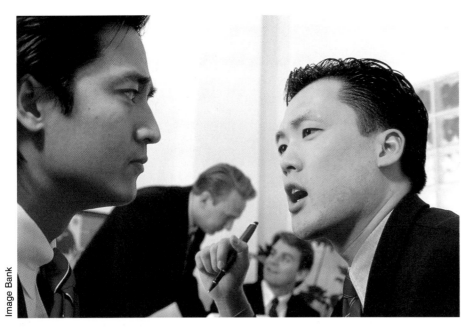

Image Bank

For optimum performance in business activities, such as important meetings, it is wise to choose days when the intellectual and emotional cycles are at their peak.

Who discovered biorhythms?

Three people were separately responsible for the discovery of biorhythms: a psychologist, a doctor, and an engineer. The psychologist was Professor Hermann Swoboda of the University of Vienna. Shortly before the end of the 19th century, Swoboda became aware that there was a repetitive pattern in the behavior of human beings. He continued his research into this pattern and was able to chart a physical cycle lasting 23 days that affected a person's physical abilities and reactions.

Swoboda also noticed a 28-day cycle governing the emotions. This sometimes coincided with the menstrual cycle in women, making it easy to confuse the two. However, he was able to establish that this emotional cycle was separate from the menstrual cycle because it occurred in men, too. When he was convinced that his findings were accurate, Swoboda published his first book, *Periodicity in Man's Life*.

By coincidence, a Berlin nose-and-throat specialist, Wilhelm Fliess, was making similar discoveries at the same time as Swoboda. He, too, noticed repeating patterns over 23 and 28 days—the physical and emotional cycles.

About 20 years after Swoboda and Fliess, Professor Alfred Teltscher, an engineer and student of mathematics, became intrigued by the possibility of an intellectual cycle. Teltscher had become aware that individual people showed varying intellectual abilities at different times. On

one day, a particular person would grasp new ideas easily and would be able to think clearly and reason well. On another day, the very same person would have difficulty with intellectual tasks. Teltscher investigated further and discovered that these fluctuations in ability formed a pattern spread over a period of 33 days—the intellectual cycle.

Two doctors at Pennsylvania University, Rexford Hersey and Michael John Bennett, who were working independently of Teltscher, confirmed his findings.

How biorhythms work

Biorhythms have been compared to astrology. However, astrology is based on a belief that human beings are influenced by the position of the stars and planets in relation to each other. In biorhythms, the influence comes from a person's own internal rhythms, not external forces.

The three biorhythms are said to begin at birth and continue rising and falling throughout a lifetime. They can be plotted on a graph representing a particular stretch of time, say a month. Such a graph is called a biogram. Looking at it allows a person to anticipate favorable and less favorable days in the near future.

If a biogram covers one month, it would be divided up vertically into the number of days in that month. It would also be divided horizontally by a line across the center. The "waves" of each cycle rise above, cross, and fall below the "horizon line" in an endlessly repeating pattern.

The first half of each cycle begins with a rising wave: this is the active, energy-packed phase. A person will reach the peak of their powers on the crest of the wave, the highest point, halfway through the first half of the cycle. After this, their

Planning your own biogram

1 Calculate the total number of days in your life so far, starting from the day of your birth. Remember to include an extra day for each leap year (do not just add an extra day for every four years; you will need to check when the last leap year was and count backward from there to get the total number to date).
2 Divide the total number of days in your life by the number of days in each cycle. If there are any days left over, this will show you which day you are on in that cycle now. If there are no days left over, you are at the beginning of a new cycle.
3 Draw up a chart. Divide it into narrow columns for the days, with a horizontal line across the center. Using a different color for each cycle, plot all three, showing where they peak, where they cross the line, and where they are at their lowest point. By comparing your biorhythms laid out in this way, you will be able to see what your energies and capabilities will be on any one day.

energies and abilities will gradually diminish as the wave falls below the horizon and passes into the second half of the cycle. This is the passive phase, when energy is being restored in preparation for the next active period.

Critical days

Surprisingly the most unstable time in each cycle is not the lowest point in the passive phase but the day on which the cycle crosses the dividing line between its active and passive halves—like an engine changing from one gear to another. It is at such sensitive turning points that a person is more likely to make mistakes, have accidents, or behave in an uncharacteristic way because they are physically, emotionally, or mentally off-kilter. The days when these gear changes occur are called critical days. The effects of a critical day can last between 24 and 48 hours.

Each cycle has two such days—one at the beginning and one in the middle. There is also a third critical day as one cycle ends and another one begins. In the 23-day physical cycle, the critical days fall on the first and 12th days, with the next cycle beginning on day 24. In the 28-day emotional cycle, the first and 15th are the critical days, and the next cycle starts on day 29. In the 33-day intellectual cycle, the first and 17th are critical days, and the next cycle begins on day 34.

Sample biorhythm chart for 33-day period

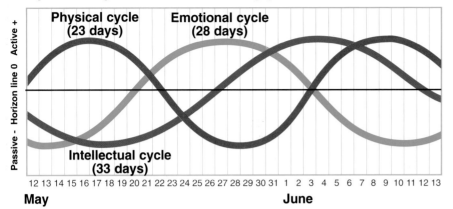

very first physical cycle will end when a baby is 23 days old, the first emotional cycle at 28 days of age, and the first intellectual cycle at 33 days.

The three rhythms continue rising and falling throughout life, beginning and ending at different times. There is one point, however, when they do coincide once more, as they did when someone was born. This "grand triple critical day" when all three cycles start together again has been calculated to fall 21,252 days after birth, or at 58.2 years of age. Up to this moment, a person will have experienced 924 physical cycles, 759 emotional cycles, and 644 intellectual cycles.

Biorhythms in action

Biorhythms have no effect on the external conditions and events in a person's life, as the planets and stars of astrology are said to do. What they do affect, however, is the way in which someone reacts to those conditions and events. Of course, different reactions produce different outcomes, so in one sense,

In addition to these critical days, there are other times that are less troublesome but still need to be guarded against. These are the days when a particular cycle is either at its peak or its lowest point. On peak days, a person may have an excess of energy in one area so that they become overconfident and go overboard. On days when the passive phase is at its lowest, the opposite is true and a person will be least effective physically or mentally, or at their most negative emotionally. The physical cycle peaks around day 7 and is at its lowest around day 18. The emotional cycle peaks around day 8 and has its lowest point around day 22. The intellectual cycle peaks at about day 9 and is at its lowest around day 26.

In any one month, there are at least six critical days in everyone's biorhythms. Out of an average month of 30 days, these six days represent one-fifth or 20 percent, which means that people are in a critical phase of some kind for at least 20 percent of their lives. In the case of a 30-year-old woman, for example, she would have had a minimum of at least six whole years in her life of being particularly off-kilter physically, emotionally, and mentally.

Double and triple critical days

Because there are three separate biorhythms operating in any one person at the same time, this means that two or even three critical days from different cycles can sometimes coincide. On a double critical day in, say, both the emotional and physical cycles, an individual who is normally calm may flare up in an angry show of emotion and may express their feelings physically by throwing or breaking things or even lashing out at another person. On a triple critical day, when the intellectual cycle is also at one

The three biorhythm cycles all begin simultaneously at birth, but quickly fall out of sync with each other. Like the phases of the moon, the patterns are unchangeable.

of its turning points, the potential for uncharacteristic behavior is multiplied by three times.

Although the three biorhythms all begin at the same time at the moment when a person is born, they soon fall out of step with each other because they each last for different lengths of time. The

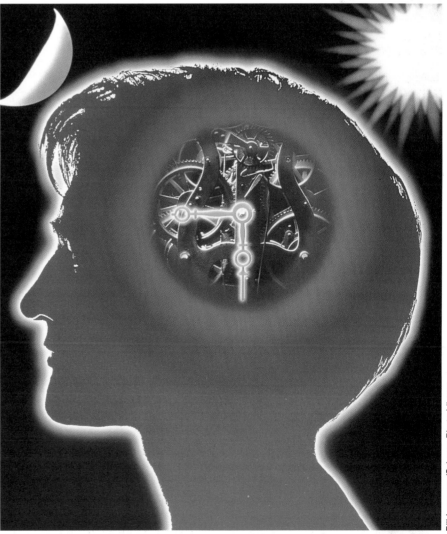

BIORHYTHMS

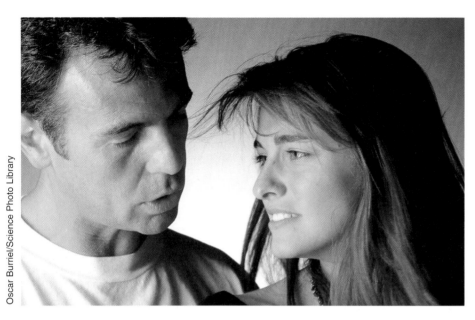

Oscar Burriel/Science Photo Library

biorhythms can be said to have an indirect effect on a person's fortunes. For example, if someone has to go for a job interview, they should choose a time when they will be in a positive frame of mind, both emotionally and intellectually. If the date suggested for the interview happens to coincide with a critical day in either of these cycles, another date could be fixed during a more favorable phase.

Knowing in advance where active and passive phases and critical days are going to fall enables a person to make allowances for their behavior. For example, a student may use exactly the same route and method of transportation to get to college every day. During the active physical phase, the journey will seem easy and effortless, and the student will arrive at the destination full of energy for the day to come. However, as the cycle passes into its negative phase, making the journey to college will become unbearable, and just getting through the day will seem a struggle. Here, there has been no change in external circumstances—what has changed is the person's reactions, under the influence of biorhythms.

Critical days in the physical cycle might lead to accidents, such as pulling a muscle while playing tennis, due to misjudgment of physical abilities on that day.

The active phase of the emotional cycle brings a sense of friendliness and optimism, which makes it a good time for socializing and mixing with other people. As the cycle moves into its negative phase, however, those same friends, family, and coworkers may suddenly become a source of irritation. Under the biorhythm's negative influence, a person may feel depressed and be hurt or angered by words or actions that would not normally bother them.

The positive phase of the intellectual cycle is a good time for mental work of all kinds—writing essays or reports, studying, having discussions, working out a spending budget, starting a new job. During the negative phase of this cycle, a person's ability to learn, understand, and concentrate will be lowered, and even the easiest mental task may seem difficult. This is the time to review work already done, not to begin something new.

Statistical evidence

In 1939 Dr. Hans Schwing of the Swiss Federal Institute of Technology published a study based on biorhythms and their effects on accidents and accidental deaths. For his study, Dr. Schwing used two sets of figures. The first were a number of cases kept on record in the city of Zurich: of these, 700 were accident cases and 300 were cases of accidental death. The second statistic he used was the total biorhythmic span of 21,252 days (the time it takes for all three cycles to coincide again). Out of this figure, 16,925 days, or 79.6 percent of the total, were noncritical days, and 4,327 days, or 20.4 percent, were critical days.

When Schwing compared the two sets of figures, he discovered an interesting ratio: nearly 60 percent of the accidents had occurred in the 20.4 percent of critical days, while only 40 percent had occurred in the remaining 79.6 percent of the time. So, over half the accidents had taken place in only a fifth of the time. Equally astonishing findings were published in 1954 by Rheinhold Bochow at the Humbold University in Berlin. This report was based on a study of 497 accidents that had involved agricultural machinery. Only 2.2 percent of accidents fell on noncritical, mixed-rhythm days,

but a staggering total of 97.85 percent occurred on critical days—with 46.5 percent on double critical days.

Police records also suggest some interesting connections between biorhythms and crime. In the intellectual cycle, a crime is 4.7 percent more likely to be committed during the negative phase than the positive one. Violent crimes, such as murder or armed robbery, appear to be more frequent when a criminal has been in a positive physical phase, with large amounts of physical energy, and negative emotional and intellectual phases.

Several American airline companies have also taken biorhythms seriously and have used them as a tool in planning the work schedules of their pilots and air-traffic controllers.

Birth

Childbirth is one of the most rewarding experiences in a woman's life, and if she is well informed about what is involved, she will be confident and relaxed during labor and the birth itself.

Q Is it true that if I eat well in pregnancy I will have an easier labor?

A It is true that women who are fit and healthy when labor begins are likely to cope better. Eating a balanced diet, in addition to avoiding cigarettes and alcohol, is known to result in healthier babies. If a mother and baby are healthy, there is less chance of complications arising. But there is no need to eat for two.

Q What can I do to make my labor as easy as possible? I feel nervous about it, and I want to take every precaution.

A It helps to understand what is happening to your body in labor. Women who are afraid of birth are usually very tense. In extreme cases, tension can slow labor, and a prolonged labor is more tiring. Most hospitals provide some prenatal education. Even if it is only parent skills, it will include information about what will happen in labor. Other hospitals or health clinics offer classes in relaxation (psychoprophylaxis) that are invaluable in making labor as easy as possible.

Q My sister has told me about natural childbirth. She gave birth naturally in a special clinic. Can I have it in the hospital? I would also like my husband to stay with me. Will the hospital allow this?

A Most women will have a natural birth wherever they are. In the hospital, however, a number of aids to birth are used— such as the monitoring machine— which can also be seen as interference. While it is true that a lot of hospital procedures are unnecessary in normal labor, they are carried out to prevent complications. It is the duty of the hospital to prevent anything from going wrong, but there is no harm in asking firmly why each procedure is to be done and if it is necessary for you. No procedure in normal labor will warrant your husband's absence, but discuss this with your doctor ahead of time.

Having a baby usually means going into the hospital, particularly if it is a first baby. Although giving birth almost always has nothing to do with ill health, going into the hospital, where specialists are always available, is advised in most cases, just in case a problem or unexpected complication should arise during labor or immediately after birth.

Of course most women are unlikely to have any problems and will enjoy a healthy pregnancy and normal labor. And a woman does have the right to choose where her baby will be born, so if having a baby at home is desired, it can usually be arranged.

However, women giving birth in the hospital, especially for the first time, will find it helpful and reassuring to know exactly what happens and what to expect—and so will their partners.

A very special experience

Having a baby is a perfectly natural process. A baby is born practically every second somewhere in the world. At the same time, it is an amazing experience for those involved. This is because every human being is unique, and every birth a very special experience.

No one can predict what will happen during labor, but obstetricians—doctors who specialize in the delivery of babies—nurses, and nurse-midwives are able to recognize when things may go wrong and can deal with the unexpected with the maximum degree of safety for the mother and her baby. Deaths are now rare in childbirth. Old wives' tales, superstitions, and ancient folklore concerning birth can be explained away.

The start of labor

No one really knows how labor begins, but there are a number of theories. The most recent is that the hormone levels in the baby change, triggering labor. Labor can begin in one of three ways. In the last

Even immediately after birth, the baby's flexing and grasping movements are already strongly developed.

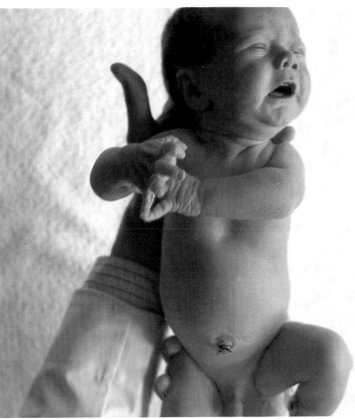

Shaun Skelly/MC Library

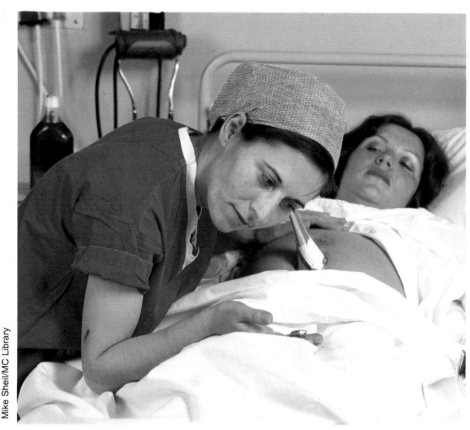

Mike Sheil/MC Library

One of the routine tests carried out on admission to the hospital is a check of the baby's heartbeat.

months of pregnancy, the uterus (womb) prepares for birth with a tightening and relaxing of its muscles, known as Braxton Hicks contractions. When the tightenings become regular and strong, and last for more than just a few seconds, true labor has generally begun.

Contractions occur every 10 to 15 minutes, and they remain constant; if they become irregular, it may be a false alarm, and be more Braxton Hicks contractions. This is why it is important not to rush to the hospital.

Signs to watch for
When the baby is due to be born, a woman may notice a small discharge of blood and mucus from her vagina when she visits the bathroom, or she may simply find a slight discharge of mucus coming from the vagina. This can occur by itself, followed a little later by contractions. It is usually a sign that labor has begun, for the mucus acts as a plug over the cervix (neck of the uterus). As the uterus opens up, this plug is released from the cervix.

It is common for contractions to begin very soon after the discharge. If the contractions start first, the discharge often follows. Some women do not notice the

discharge at all, especially if it is not bloodstained. (Bleeding with contractions is not normal, and in cases of slight bleeding the doctor should be called at once and asked for advice. With severe bleeding, the woman should go to the hospital immediately.)

The third way labor may begin is with the breaking of the water—the rupturing of the membranes of the amniotic sac that protects the baby in the uterus. In most cases, contractions will soon follow. Occasionally, however, the water breaks and nothing happens. In this case, the baby is no longer protected from infection and the woman should contact the hospital immediately.

The obstetrician may, for a number of different reasons, decide to speed things up, in which case he or she administers a drug that stimulates the uterus and causes contractions. If this is done after labor has started, it is called an accelerated labor. When it is done to start labor, usually in conjunction with the artificial rupture of the membranes, it is called induced labor.

When to go to the hospital
If there are no complications, home is the best and most comfortable place to be in early labor. It is extremely rare for a baby to be born within the first hour after the onset of labor. If it is a first baby, labor may last about 12 hours; if it is a second or subsequent baby, it is possible that labor will be quicker, lasting about seven hours, but these times are averages and and can vary enormously.

If a woman is able to relax at home between contractions, she can make last-minute preparations then. It is best to eat something; but if she cannot face food, a hot, sweet drink will prevent the blood sugar from dropping (which will make her feel tired) as labor progresses.

Pain relief in labor

- Relaxation techniques (psycho-prophylaxis) are very helpful. Ask your doctor if there are any classes you can attend
- Meperidine hydrochloride (Demerol) is the drug most commonly used for relieving the pain of contractions during the first and second stages of labor. This synthetic opiate acts mainly on the central nervous system and is usually administered by intramuscular injection. Since meperidine crosses the placental barrier, it may cause depressed or delayed respiration in the newborn infant. These effects may be less if there is under an hour between injection of the drug and delivery
- Other drugs are sometimes given during labor in conjunction with the primary analgesic. These include a tranquilizer, such as promethazine hydrochloride (Phenergan); a barbiturate, such as secobarbital

(Seconal) or pentobarbital (Nembutal); or an amnesiac, such as scopolamine
- An epidural injection involves injecting a local anesthetic into the epidural space (just in front of the spinal cord). A fine needle with a plastic tube inside is placed in the middle of the back. Once the tube is inserted, the drug is given. The area below will be numbed so that contractions are not felt. This drug is very effective, and frequent doses can be given without disturbing the mother. It may cause a drop in blood pressure or other minor reactions such as shivering or faintness, but an intravenous drip is always used to counteract these symptoms. Sometimes the woman's ability to push the baby out is reduced because the pushing sensation is lost. A forceps delivery may be necessary. The anesthetic can cause the baby to be drowsy at birth

The labor ward staff can be kept informed by phone about the progress of the labor, and they will tell a woman when to come into the hospital. If she is anxious, she may prefer to go in just in case, but there is usually no need to hurry.

Arrival at the hospital

The labor ward in a small hospital is often separate from the admission ward, and a woman may not see it until she goes into the second stage of labor. In larger, more modern units, the labor wards consist of admission rooms, first-stage rooms, and delivery suites.

On admission, a woman will be asked for details, including a history of her labor up to that point. A vaginal examination (internal) will normally be carried out to confirm the onset of labor by checking for the dilation of the cervix (opening of the neck of the uterus). Someone will check the position of the baby, the baby's heartbeat, and perform several other routine observations that are designed to prevent any complications at an early stage and also to improve the mother's personal comfort.

Routine tests

Tests will include a check on blood pressure, pulse, temperature, and the length of the contractions. A sample of urine will also be tested to show if the blood-sugar level is satisfactory. Sometimes in labor the blood-sugar level drops, and sugar water is given to prevent exhaustion. Some hospitals do not allow a woman to eat or drink while in labor, not just because some women may vomit, but because if there are problems that require a general anesthetic, the stomach must be empty.

Coping with an emergency delivery

Sometimes a baby is born very quickly. This may happen before medical help can be called. It is vital that any helper should know what to do in this situation.

- It should be remembered that a fast labor is generally a normal labor, and the mother should be reminded of this to reassure her
- Cleanliness is essential. The helper must scrub his or her hands thoroughly
- The first stage of labor usually lasts several hours, but it can also be surprisingly brief. The mother should try to relax without worrying between contractions. She should use the bathroom and not be alarmed if there is a small discharge of blood. This is quite normal
- The second stage of labor lasts until the birth. The mother should lie on her back with knees bent up and feet apart. She should push with each contraction, relaxing in between
- At the beginning of each contraction, a deep breath should be taken and released, and then another breath taken, which should be held while the contraction lasts. This helps ease the contractions and provides the baby with oxygen via the mother's bloodstream
- During the first or second stage of labor, there will be a sudden discharge of watery fluid from the vagina—this is from the bag of water that protects the baby in the womb and is completely normal
- The baby is generally born headfirst, and as it emerges, the mother should pant. This helps stop violent contractions that would push the baby out too fast
- The helper should now support the baby's head using the palms of the hands, and when the shoulders emerge, lift the baby out by holding it under the armpits. The baby should be put on the mother's stomach. The umbilical cord may be cut with sterile scissors and a knot tied in it to prevent bleeding—but this can be left until help arrives
- If the baby is breast-fed straight after birth, the afterbirth (the placenta and fetal membranes) will be expelled naturally, because breast-feeding releases a hormone that stimulates the process

---

It used to be common practice in hospitals for a woman to be given a warm enema (to clear the back passage of feces); this is sometimes still done if necessary. Occasionally the pubic hair is shaved to reduce chances of infection.

Monitoring the birth

It is also usual in large maternity units for women in labor to be monitored. This means wearing a rubber belt around the abdomen that has a large knob on the top attached by wires to a machine. The machine records when the contractions begin, when they peak, and when they end. (The doctor or nurse will still feel for the contractions at certain intervals.)

Monitoring does not mean there is something wrong. It is simply a way of saving work for the nurse or doctor by providing a constant check on what is happening to mother and baby.

The progress of labor

To check the progress of labor, a woman will usually be given an internal examination every three or four hours, depending on her individual progress. On one of these occasions, a tiny clip may be attached to the baby's scalp and then to the monitoring machine so that the heart rate can be recorded.

If labor progresses normally and there are no complications, routine observations and monitor recordings will continue with no other interferences, except perhaps for an injection of glucose to keep the blood sugar level up and prevent exhaustion. If the woman decides she would like an epidural or a local anesthetic to prevent the pain, the obstetrician or anesthetist may give her one.

If labor is progressing well—most hospitals have a graph that maps out what

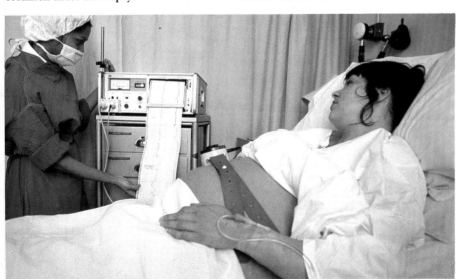

A monitoring machine can be used to record the contractions and thereby check the *progress of labor. It also permits the woman to watch each contraction.*

the normal progress should be—and the waters are still intact, they will not be broken artificially since this will eventually happen automatically. Occasionally labor slows down and the waters will be broken artificially to speed it up again. This is a fairly painless procedure.

End of the first stage

Toward the end of the first stage of labor, the woman will find that the contractions begin to get much closer together and that they can be very strong. Labor is now fully established and the baby is nearly ready to be born.

This transition period is recognized as a sign that the cervix is more or less fully dilated (usually around 4 in, or 9–10 cm). A positive sign that the cervix is ready is the gaping of the anus as the head of the baby arrives at the perineum—the area between the anus and the vagina. This area thins and bulges out as the head descends. The woman will feel a very

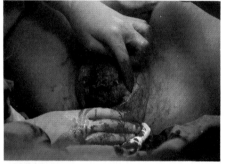

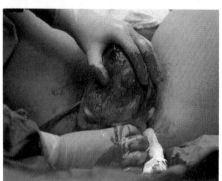

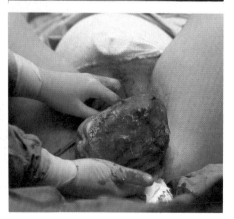

strong urge to push the baby out but may be told to wait a bit if the cervix is not fully dilated.

The second stage of labor

This is when the cervix is fully dilated and the pushing can start. It is now that husbands and partners can be most useful in encouraging the mother-to-be. It is the end of labor, she is tired, and some really hard work is yet to come. Coping with those very strong contractions in the late stages of labor may seem almost unbearable, but when pushing begins, it is a relief—all the woman's energy goes into the pushing, the labor feels as if it is progressing, and the contractions do not seem too strong after all.

The urge to push is normally a natural reaction, but if an epidural is being used, the woman may not get this sensation and will need extra help. As the baby's head descends, the perineum will stretch. The doctor or nurse-midwife controls the head as it emerges to prevent the perineum from tearing.

If the perineum is too thin and is therefore in danger of severe tearing, or if the baby is distressed and needs to be delivered quickly, then the area will be cut with special scissors. This is called an episiotomy and is less painful than one might expect. But most women will stretch adequately without any tearing.

As the baby's shoulders emerge, the birth process is almost at an end. In an ideal situation, the baby should then be lifted onto the mother's stomach while the umbilical cord is cut and a piece of thread tied around the cut ends to stop the bleeding. Providing the room is warm and all is well, there is no reason for the baby to be taken away for measurements and tests immediately—allowing time for the bonding between mother and child to begin.

The baby is actually born during the second stage of labor, with the head emerging first, followed by the shoulders. After this, the body slides out easily.

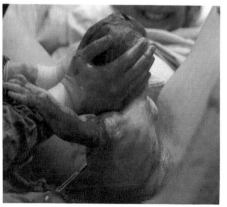

The first moments

Holding the baby as soon as possible is very important. Research shows that mothers who cuddle and fondle their babies from birth are more likely to make early, close relationships with them. This process is called bonding. This, of course, does not mean that if a baby is taken from its mother at birth their relationship is permanently harmed—bonding can take place later.

Before the first stage of labor, the baby's head rests on the neck of the uterus.

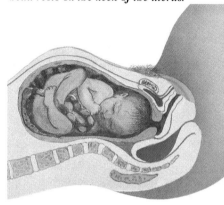

Contractions during the first stages are aimed at dilating the neck of the uterus.

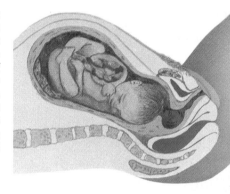

With its head past the neck of the uterus, the baby twists to allow the body to emerge.

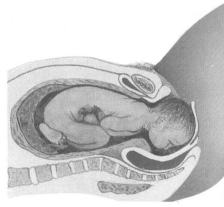

Some women do not possess an inborn maternal instinct, and it is these who may find it more difficult to attach themselves to their babies once they have given birth. But most women gradually grow to love their babies over several months.

The third stage of labor
During the third stage of labor, the afterbirth is delivered. Immediately after the birth of the baby, the muscles of the uterus relax. Within minutes, contractions resume; these serve to separate the placenta from the uterine wall and then expel it. A woman may be unaware of this because the birth area is numb for a while after the delivery of the baby. The delivery of the placenta is painless and over quickly.

The doctor or nurse-midwife will gently pull on the cord to ease the placenta out. This process takes from about three to 10 minutes. When it is left to be expelled without help, the process is usually a little longer, lasting from about 20 minutes to an hour. If necessary, a drug may be given to help this process.

If the mother puts the baby to the breast immediately after it is born, a

The baby emerges, to be placed immediately on his mother's abdomen. The umbilical cord, linking the blood supplies of mother and child, is still attached. This cord, which will now be cut, is about 20 in (50 cm) long and thicker than a finger.

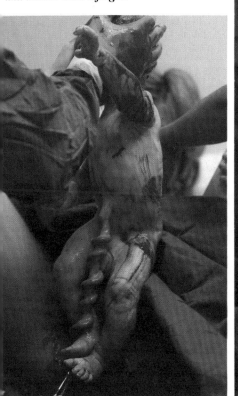

hormone will be released that will cause the uterus to contract and expel the placenta more rapidly.

Caesarean section
The normal process of labor may be bypassed, where necessary, by a Caesarean section. This is an abdominal operation where the baby is born through an incision, either in an emergency, when the lives of the baby and/or mother are at risk, or as a planned procedure for those women who are known to have complications that would prevent them from having a normal birth.

A Caesarean section may be necessary, for example, if the baby is in distress. Distress can be detected by the doctor or nurse-midwife from the baby's heartbeat pattern, from hypoxia (a lack of oxygen in the baby's bloodstream), or from the release of meconium (a green-black substance) from its bowels. The umbilical cord may become wrapped around the

baby's neck, or its head may be tipped so that it cannot fit through the birth canal.

Births requiring an emergency Caesarean are very rare, however. Most problems that occur can be handled easily by a doctor or a nurse-midwife in a hospital setting.

There are also a few nonemergency situations that call for a Caesarean section. Some women, for example, have a small pelvic canal, or the afterbirth may have become embedded and be likely to bleed. Breech babies (where a part of the body other than the head is born first) are sometimes delivered by Caesarean.

The baby can be breast-fed normally after a Caesarean section. But a period of convalescence is required for the mother, as with other operations.

Complete safety
Having a baby today is considered a completely safe experience. When everything goes well, there is no need for medical

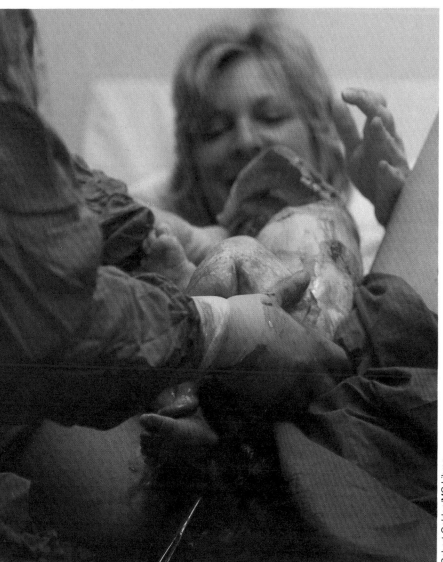

Q What will happen if I go into labor early?

A If the baby is very tiny, then all efforts will be made to delay the progress of labor, and hopefully stop it altogether. There are special drugs that can be given to relax the uterus. If this method does not succeed, then labor will progress and all precautions will be taken for the birth of a premature baby. A pediatrician (a doctor specializing in problems of babies and children) will attend the labor and will probably put the baby in an incubator in the intensive care nursery for observation and possible treatment. Abnormally small babies are vulnerable, and it is much better if the pregnancy goes to its full term. But most survive to grow up healthy.

Q What will happen if I go past my delivery date?

A It is very rare indeed for a baby to die just because it is overdue. If labor does not start of its own accord, it can be induced with a drug. The water will also be broken artificially. It is difficult to be totally accurate over dates, and for this reason, some women will go beyond the time predicted for the delivery by as long as three weeks with no danger to themselves or the baby.

Q Is it true that the birth of my second baby will be easier than the first?

A Every labor is different and every baby is unique. But in a second labor, the muscles will have already been stretched and the labor is often quicker, especially the second stage. But this does not necessarily mean it will be easier.

Q I am expecting twins. Will the labor be more difficult than with a single baby?

A Not necessarily, but it may be a little longer than average. One possible problem is that the babies may be born early because of the extra weight on the neck of the uterus. If there is a risk of them being premature, they may require special attention at the hospital, both before and after birth.

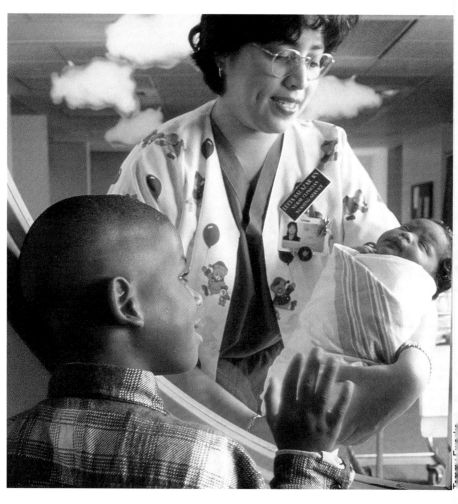

interference, and many hospitals will respect a couple's wishes for as natural a delivery as possible. However, sometimes things go wrong, and what may have seemed a normal labor turns out to be not so simple. A nurse-midwife is trained to recognize signs that show the labor is becoming complicated, and when she detects them, to call for a doctor. In a hospital, this help is immediately available. All obstetric units have obstetricians on call who frequently check up on normal deliveries and attend abnormal ones.

Giving birth at home
A home birth can be arranged provided there is no likelihood of risk to mother or baby and as long as the mother has no history of difficult pregnancies. The prenatal examinations may be carried out by the nurse-midwife and the doctor, and it is a good idea for the mother-to-be to seek their support for her decision.

Contact with the local hospital's maternity department is important and should be kept up during pregnancy so that it will not be too unsettling if hospitalization is required at the last moment. The nurse-midwife will give advice on getting the home ready for a delivery.

The arrival of a new baby is an exciting event in the life of the whole family, including older brothers and sisters, who will be keen to meet the new arrival.

Since childbirth is a bit messy, any furniture near the birth area should be covered with paper or plastic sheeting. Good lighting and heating are essential, with a bright overhead light and another lamp by the bed. Constant, safe heat of around 68°F (20°C) is necessary, since newborn babies lose heat very rapidly.

The nurse-midwife will stay with the mother throughout labor, at the birth of the baby, and during the third stage when the placenta is expelled. The doctor may make periodic checks and will certainly want to be there at the delivery. If the husband or partner is able to be present at the birth, he can offer a great deal of support to his partner, and he will not feel left out of the experience. Most labor procedures will be the same as in a hospital, except that there are not as many painkilling drugs available. A great advantage of a home birth is that, in the familiar surroundings of her own home, a woman should be more relaxed, and thus find labor easier.

Birthmarks

Q I am expecting a baby and have heard that birthmarks can sometimes be caused by the mother receiving a shock during her pregnancy. Is this true, and can I do anything to avoid getting a shock?

A No—this is an old wives' tale that attempted to find a cause for birthmarks. There is no evidence at all that birthmarks are caused by any external influence during pregnancy, be it emotional or physical.

Q Can my baby's strawberry birthmark lead to side effects or complications?

A The strawberry mark is one of the most common birthmarks and may become sore and ulcerated, but this can be prevented by carefully washing and powdering it.

Q If I have a difficult labor and birth, will it give my baby birthmarks?

A No—birthmarks are not caused by problems during labor. There may be some bruising or dimpling of the skin if forceps are used for a difficult delivery, but this will soon fade and it should not be confused with a true birthmark.

Q Can birthmarks disappear by themselves?

A The strawberry mark and another common blemish, known as the stork mark, usually fade, but other types tend to be more permanent.

Q Is it true that moles can be malignant?

A A few moles can be malignant or may eventually become so. Signs that a mole is malignant are: sudden increase in size; bleeding; continuous itching; development of further moles nearby; and a darkening in color. If you suspect a mole of being malignant, see a doctor immediately. Removal of the mole usually cures the problem, but any delay may be dangerous.

Many old wives' tales claim to explain why birthmarks appear, but, in fact, they have no known cause. All but a few are harmless, and most can be treated or removed.

The term *birthmark* is used to describe any noticeable abnormality, such as a pit, a swelling, or a mark on the skin of a baby. It may be present at birth or appear soon after.

Such marks can be thought of as defects in the development of part of the skin and consist of either groups of abnormal blood vessels, collections of cells responsible for the production of pigment (coloring), or groups of cells responsible for the formation of the surface of skin, properly called the epidermis. The usual word used by doctors to describe one of these marks is a *nevus*, or if there are more than one, *nevi*.

Birthmarks composed of abnormal blood vessels are called vascular nevi; those with pigmented cells, melanocytic nevi (or moles); and those from the epidermis, epidermal nevi.

Causes

The majority of birthmarks have no known cause, unlike those birth defects that are caused by the mother catching an infection such as rubella (German measles; see Rubella) during pregnancy. There is therefore no way to prevent a baby being born with one.

Vascular nevi

There are two types of vascular birthmarks. One, known as nevus flammeus, consists of a defect in the smallest blood vessels in the top layer of the skin. The blood vessels dilate—or widen—and this causes the redness of the overlying skin. Varieties of this type of birthmark include the salmon patch, the stork mark, the port-wine stain, and the capillary nevus.

The other type of vascular nevus is derived from patches of primitive tissue from which blood vessels are formed. When it is present after birth, it is the blemish known as a strawberry mark or cavernous nevus.

Salmon patches or stork marks are visible at birth. These birthmarks are pale pink, with fine blood vessels visible within them, and are most commonly seen on the nape of the neck, on the midforehead, and on the eyelids. The majority of them fade rapidly, and most have gone by the age of one year. They rarely, if ever, need treatment.

Mongolian spots are blue-black marks between 0.75 and 3 in (2–8 cm) that appear on the buttocks and backs of some African American, Native American, southern European, and Oriental babies. They are caused by a local accumulation of the normal skin pigment and usually

Port-wine stains can appear anywhere on the body but are most common on the face and upper body. They can measure several inches across.

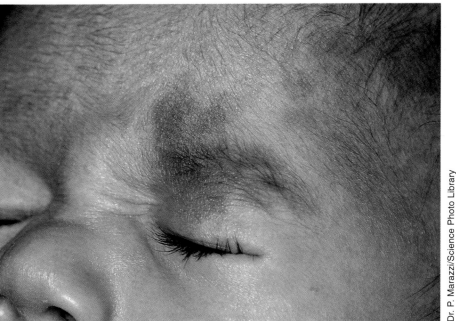

Dr. P. Marazzi/Science Photo Library

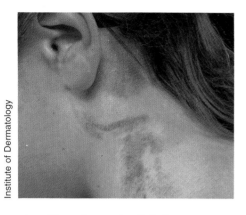

An epidermal nevus is a light brown or skin-colored permanent stain.

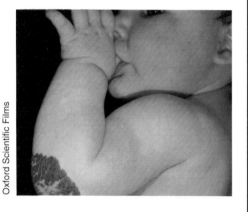

A strawberry mark is largest at nine months and then usually fades.

Birthmarks

Type	Temporary or permanent	Treatment
Salmon patch (small pink mark)	Usually fade rapidly and disappear by the age of one	Rarely need treatment
Stork mark (red mark)	Usually fade rapidly and disappear by the age of one	Rarely need treatment
Port-wine stain (large red patch, often on face)	Remain indefinitely	Cosmetic camouflage Can be cut out, but may require skin graft Laser treatment Occasionally tattooing Freezing
Capillary nevus (red stain under skin, caused by small blood vessels)	Permanent	Cosmetic camouflage Carbon dioxide snow (very cold, semisolid carbon dioxide) may be used to destroy small ones by freezing; large ones may be cut out Radium therapy
Strawberry mark	Usually temporary	90 percent disappear without treatment Occasionally steroid drugs are prescribed
Café-au-lait patch	Remain indefinitely	Not necessary
Moles	Usually develop in childhood and adolescence; occasionally malignant and unless removed are permanent. Rarely occur on babies, but if present, have small risk of being malignant	Large ones should be removed. Moles that develop later in childhood do not usually require treatment; if they enlarge, they should be removed
Epidermal nevus	Present at birth or soon after; permanent	Can be cut out, but sometimes return Freezing effective in some cases

disappear during early childhood, around the age of four.

Port-wine stains are less common than salmon patches, but are usually permanent. They occur on any part of the body, but are most common on the face and upper part of the trunk. They range in color from pale pink to deep red or purple and can vary in size from a fraction of an inch to several inches across.

Treatment

In the case of port-wine stains, treatment is generally satisfactory. If the blemish is small enough to be completely cut out without the need for a skin graft, then a good result is assured. But if a skin graft is necessary, scarring usually occurs, which can be unsightly, and the best treatment is to hide it with makeup.

Occasionally tattooing (see Tattooing) can be used to improve the color match with the surrounding normal skin, and freezing the skin and laser treatment have been used with some success.

Lesser problems

Strawberry marks are found on up to 10 percent of babies but they are rarely visible at birth. They usually appear as red blemishes during the first month of life and can be found on any part of the body, but most often on the head and neck. They grow to reach maximum size by six to nine months and are clearly defined, domed swellings, bright pink in color.

Strawberry marks vary in size, the most common being 1-2 in (2.5-5 cm) across, but in rare cases, it can be very large. If the birthmark is located near the mouth, it may cause feeding difficulties, and if it lies near the eyes, it can cause problems with vision. But very few strawberry marks cause any complications, and at least 90 percent disappear during early childhood.

Pigmented birthmarks

Pigmented birthmarks include café-au-lait patches—flat, pale-brown marks, 2-8 in (5-20 cm) across—and moles. Café-au-lait patches, which occur in up to 10 percent of babies, usually appear on the trunk and are not very noticeable.

Moles are collections of pigment cells—those which give the skin color. Uncommon in babyhood, they are more common in childhood and adolescence. When present at birth, they have a small risk of becoming malignant. Moles that develop later on in childhood have little risk of malignancy and can be cut out under local anesthetic if necessary.

Bites and stings

Q Is it all right if I take an aspirin or other form of painkiller for pain relief after being stung by a wasp?

A Aspirin and other forms of painkiller won't do any harm, but local remedies, such as a soothing ointment, would probably relieve the pain better. The pain should soon go away.

Q How can I tell the difference between a bee sting and a wasp sting?

A The best method is to find the insect itself, which has probably died after stinging in self-defense. If this is impossible, remember that a wound with a sting remaining inside it is more likely to be a bee sting. If you have no idea whether the insect was a bee, a wasp, or indeed anything else, it is a good idea to apply a cold compress followed by antihistamine cream. If you are in real discomfort, or if the discomfort lasts for some time, see your doctor for advice and treatment.

Q My son was bitten by a neighbor's dog. Should I take him to the doctor?

A Animal bites should be seen by a doctor if the skin is broken. With a severe cut, stitches may be needed. However, if the skin is unbroken after a bite, cleaning the skin and applying soothing ointment are all that is necessary, so long as no swelling or other symptoms of infection develop later.

Q When I was on vacation last year, a mosquito bite on my arm swelled into a big lump. Does this mean that I am allergic to mosquitoes?

A It may mean that the bite became infected and healed by itself or that a mild allergic reaction occurred. If you use an antihistamine cream, it will help to counteract such a reaction. Where a swelling becomes larger than expected following a bite or sting, it is always a good idea to see your doctor promptly.

Basic first aid is usually adequate for treating most bites and stings, but sometimes medical help is urgently needed.

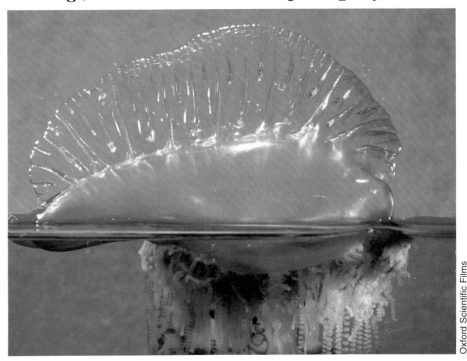

Oxford Scientific Films

The Portuguese man-of-war jellyfish gives a serious sting. Get medical help.

Many insects, some plants, and some marine creatures can sting. Many animals and insects and some reptiles can bite. In some countries, poisonous insects are dangerous. Deaths from such bites or stings are rare, but prompt action is important. The victim should be taken immediately to the nearest hospital or poison control center along with the dead insect or animal, if possible, or at least a good description of it, because this will help the doctor.

When traveling abroad, it is best to obtain information about harmful pests before going. Inoculations and other precautions must not be neglected.

Keeping pests away

The greatest risk of being bitten or stung comes from insects, such as bees or hornets; parasites, such as mosquitoes or fleas; and creatures encountered on vacation, such as venom-secreting snails and jellyfish. Keep unwanted insect visitors out by killing them on sight and maintaining a general level of cleanliness.

During hot, damp weather, when insects breed most rapidly, a hanging insecticide will kill winged insects for several months. In the backyard, a stagnant pond will attract mosquitoes—so build a pond at the furthest end of the yard, away from the house. When picnicking or sitting on the grass, always put down a groundsheet, and avoid eating sweet, sticky foods, which attract wasps. At the beach, learn to recognize stinging jellyfish and poisonous snails.

It is best not to sit too close to flowers where bees gather. A swarm of bees, wasps, or hornets should never be approached—an expert should be called.

Insects living in gardening clothes or shoes normally kept outside are a common source of stings. Shake gardening clothes and boots before putting them on, in case there is anything lurking in them.

Domestic pets

Dogs should be obedience-trained to reduce the risk of their biting people. Other people's pets should not be touched until they have had a chance to get to know you, and you, them. Children should be taught to treat all animals with caution, respect, and kindness—household pets should not be treated like toys. Mauled kittens, puppies, and even hamsters can turn into potentially dangerous biters through abuse. Special care should be taken when dealing with guard dogs, such as German shepherds, rottweilers, Doberman pinschers, and bull terriers. Children should be taught to stay away from them.

FIRST AID

Take care
Any bite or sting can lead to infection, so you must always clean the wound thoroughly. Warm water and soap make the best cleanser. If possible, the soap should not contain a detergent, perfume, or similar irritants.

After cleaning, the wound should be rinsed in clear water. If you have an antiseptic, it can now be applied. Remember to check the bottle for the correct dilutions of disinfectant or similar substances.

Cover the clean wound with a dry, sterile dressing or a laundered handkerchief. If there is increased pain and inflammation over the next day or two, infection has set in and you must see your doctor.

First-aid essentials
- Pair of fine tweezers
- Tube of antihistamine cream (such as Benadryl)
- Insect-repellent cream or spray
- Antiseptic cream
- Antiseptic liquid
- Pack of assorted-size needles to remove stings (sterilize in boiling water before use)
- Antiflea powder (safe for use with pets or children)
- Antiseptic wet-wipes for cleansing in the absence of soap and water
- Small packet of sodium bicarbonate (baking soda)
- Small bottle of vinegar (or lemon juice)
- Large sterile gauze dressing (a clean handkerchief can be substituted)
- Roll of bandage
- Assorted nonwaterproof bandages
- Calamine lotion
- Aspirin

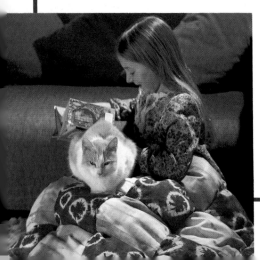

Common bites and stings

Source	Prevention	First aid	Later treatment
Jellyfish	Do not swim in water where jellyfish are known to live	Get victim to shore and pick off jellyfish tentacles with care. Cleanse sting and apply antihistamine cream	Seek medical help, especially for the sting of Portuguese man-of-war
Dog bites	Avoid strange dogs and train your own not to snap	Wash and dress the wound and see your doctor if the skin is broken	Stitches or tetanus shot. Treatment for rabies may be required
Lice	Keep hair and body clean; comb hair with a fine-tooth comb daily	For head lice, wash hair with insecticide shampoo or cream rinse. For body lice, boil linen and take daily hot baths, followed by clean clothes treated with powder	Continue treatment until all lice and nits (eggs) have vanished
Mosquitoes	Cover yourself after dark. Avoid stagnant water. Burn a mosquito stick by the bed. Apply insect repellent	Apply antihistamine cream or rubbing alcohol; cologne or cold water will do if these are not available. Repeat	Avoid scratching. Take antihistamine tablets if swelling is severe
Ants	Do not sit on uncovered grass or disturb ants' nests	Treat stings with baking-soda paste or dilute ammonia	None is usually necessary
Ticks	Check for ticks on scalp and body after walking in wooded areas. Keep dogs and cats free of ticks	If the tick is embedded in the skin, use petroleum jelly, oil, alcohol, or gasoline to loosen its grip and remove it with tweezers. Kill harvest mite ticks first with weak ammonia	Soothe tick bites with calamine lotion
Fleas	Keep dogs and cats free of fleas	Treat bites with antihistamine cream or calamine. Badly affected children should see a doctor	Use a suitable powder on animals, clothes, bedding, and cushions
Poison ivy, oak, or sumac	Teach children to recognize and avoid poisonous plants	Wash area of contact immediately with soap and water	Itchy rash may be coated with calamine or topical steroid cream from the drugstore

Problem bites and stings

Bee sting

Bee stings can cause severe pain and are among the most dangerous of stings in temperate climates. Young children, old people, and those who are prone to allergies are particularly vulnerable to unpleasant results from them.

When a bee stings the flesh, the puncture area will be surrounded by a pale area of skin, and then a reddish area, which is usually swollen into a bump. The black sting embedded in the center can often be seen. This should be scraped away or gently eased out with tweezers, without squeezing the poison sac.

A bee sting has acid venom. Once the sting has been removed and the wound cleaned, it should be treated with a paste of baking soda or diluted ammonia. If these are not available, rubbing alcohol or a cold compress can be used.

The victim should rest during treatment. Be on the lookout for signs of shock. If there are multiple bee stings, a doctor should be called immediately.

Stings in the mouth are also dangerous because they can prevent proper breathing. The patient should be given a mouthwash of one teaspoon of baking soda to a glass of water, followed by ice to suck. Then he or she should be taken to the hospital, along with the dead bee, if it can be found.

Wasp stings

When a person is stung by a wasp, the puncture may or may not contain a black sting. If the sting can be seen, it should be carefully taken out with tweezers or a sterilized needle. It should not be squeezed, because this might push the venom further into the skin. The surrounding area will be whitish, then red, and probably swollen, the same as happens with a bee sting.

Wasp stings contain alkali venom. After cleansing, the wound should be dressed with vinegar or lemon juice, because the acid content neutralizes the venom. Rubbing should be avoided.

If there is no vinegar or lemon juice available, an antihistamine cream can be used until some can be found. Then the wound can be washed and dressed again. If the swelling is severe, a cold compress can be added.

If there are multiple wasp stings and the person is in shock, the doctor must be called or the patient brought to the hospital. He or she should be put on their side and given ice to suck in the meantime. With a single wasp sting, the patient should feel better after an hour or so.

Snake bites

There are at least 20 species of venomous coral snakes and pit vipers in North America alone, while Australia is home to several varieties including the world's most poisonous snake, the inland taipan. Bites from many species are extremely dangerous, although few need be fatal if medical attention is promptly obtained.

If a person is bitten by an unidentified snake, it is best to assume that it is poisonous. First aid should include applying a broad constricting band to the bitten limb. This is not the same as a tourniquet and should be tight enough only to interfere with the venous return of blood to the heart, not with the arterial flow from the heart.

It is important to act fast in cases of snakebite. Attempting to suck out the poison may not work and time should not be spent on this. If the snake can be killed easily, it is advisable to do so, and to

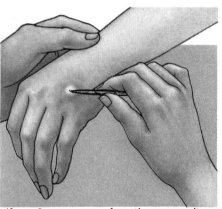

Above: Scrape away a bee sting or ease it out very gently using tweezers.
Below: Dab the area with a baking-soda paste or dilute ammonia.

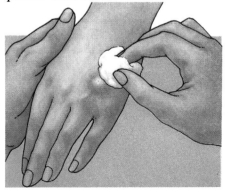

take it along to the hospital to aid in identification. However, it should be remembered that even a dead snake can reflexively inflict a venomous bite. The bitten limb should be immobilized and the victim should be transported to the hospital without delay.

Sea urchin stings

Sea urchins are found in many coastal waters and are considered tasty to eat in some countries. However, their spikes can break off in human skin, causing intense pain and the risk of infection, so it is wise to avoid swimming near them. If a sea urchin is stepped on or touched, a sharp burning pain will be felt and the area where the spine went in will be numb. The spine should be removed from the skin; it is essential to wear gloves for this or a further wound could occur. The wound should be covered with a dry dressing—a clean handkerchief will do—and a doctor seen as soon as possible.

It is necessary to see a doctor because of the high risk of infection from the sea urchin sting. The victim should be kept quiet and still during the journey to the hospital, and measures should be taken immediately if signs of shock occur.

Shock

Shock (see Shock) can result from a bite or sting where there is also a severe allergy, extreme pain, or deep emotional stress, such as fear. In most cases, shock victims recover well within an hour or so. But because shock can be dangerous, and even fatal in some cases, it is important to be able to recognize it when it occurs, and treat it correctly while waiting for the doctor.

The symptoms of shock are pale skin, restlessness, confusion, anxiety, quickened pulse, and rapid breathing. The victim may complain of thirst and may vomit, or even lose consciousness.

The treatment is to lay the victim on his or her side and stop any bleeding that would make shock worse. Tight clothing, such as collars, waistbands, and belts, should be loosened and a light blanket or overcoat put over the person. Drinks should not be given, and the victim should not be kept too warm, because warmth can make shock worse. A doctor should be seen as soon as possible.

Black eye

Q What is it about raw steak that makes it the traditional remedy for a black eye?

A A clean, raw steak provides moisture, coolness, and softness in a form that will mold itself neatly to the shape of the eye as it is pressed against it. It has no other properties to recommend it, which makes it a very expensive compress. A cloth wrung out in cold or iced water is just as good and readily available at no cost.

Q Why is a black eye the color it is, and what causes the change in color as it heals?

A When the small capillary blood vessels in the skin are broken, they leak into the surrounding tissues. They don't stay red for long, however, because they lose their oxygen and turn the blue-black color that we associate with black eyes. During recovery, the broken red cells release their hemoglobin, the pigment that originally gave them their red color. Chemical breakdown of the pigment makes the bruise change from blue-black to green-yellow, then to yellow before fading altogether as the pigment is fully absorbed by the tissues.

Q I have to go to an important formal function in five days' time. How can I disguise a black eye I received playing tennis yesterday?

A Carefully applied makeup should go a long way toward disguising it. First apply foundation in a slightly lighter color than usual to the upper and lower lid with a cosmetic sponge for an even finish. Then add powder eye shadow in a color similar to the bruising so that you can adjust the makeup on the normal eye to match. For instance, don't put violet eye shadow over green-yellow bruising. Finish with mascara.

You might also like to wear sunglasses with shaded lenses that are darker at the top than the bottom. Remember that most black eyes go away in six to eight days, so the color you will have to cover will be reduced by then.

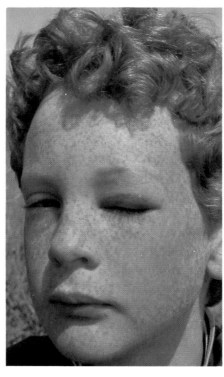

C. James Webb

A black eye may cause so much swelling that it prevents vision, but the eyeball itself is usually undamaged.

When someone has a so-called black eye, it is not the eye itself that is discolored, but the skin of the eye socket, which turns a blue-black color. The bruising can involve the upper and lower lids, and if severe, may spread onto the temples and the face. If there is a lot of swelling, the eye may also be partially or completely closed. A black eye can therefore often look very painful indeed.

Causes
Any blow to the eye socket or nose can produce a black eye. The most common causes are accidental injuries (such as walking into the corner of a cupboard door), sports injuries (particularly from boxing, but also from games such as baseball or hockey, where the injury may be from the ball or puck itself, or the bat or stick), and deliberate violence. Black eyes are also seen after any operation to the nose area—cosmetic surgery, for instance, could cause them.

Symptoms
The discoloration is the result of red blood cells being released from broken capillaries—small blood vessels—in the skin. The swelling is caused by the fluid that also leaks from capillaries.

The medical term for a black eye is *peri orbital hematoma*, which means bruising around the socket. But because the skin is tightly drawn over the eye socket the fluid and red cells have little room to move around and may slowly spread into areas beyond the eyes, such as the lids, temples, and face. The puffier the lids are the greater the chance of the eye closing through the swelling of the tissues surrounding it.

Dangers
Swelling and discoloration—and the fact that we tend to look people in the eye when we are talking to them—make a black eye look nastier than it really is. In fact, even in the event of a conjunctival hemorrhage, where some of the blood spreads into the outer covering of the eye, the eye itself is usually completely unharmed and soon returns to normal.

Nevertheless, if there is bruising of the eye, proper medical advice must be sought, especially if it has closed and the eyeball cannot be seen clearly. The doctor will check that the eye is not damaged, that the bone of the socket is not broken, and that there are no symptoms, such as a change in pupil size, which would indicate that the central nervous system is affected. Repeated black eyes may threaten the eyesight and lead to possible brain damage, which is why, nowadays, boxers are advised to spread out their matches as much as possible to give their bodies a chance to recover between fights.

Treatment
First aid aims to limit bleeding from the capillary vessels under the skin. A cold compress applied to the eye within a couple of minutes of the injury can minimize swelling and bruising, and even at a later stage, it can provide comfort. Gauze or a clear napkin or handkerchief should be soaked in cold or iced water and held against the eye.

If the compress is applied very promptly after the injury, it will limit the degree of bruising and hence the dramatic appearance of the black eye. Never use alcohol or hydrogen peroxide in the compress, in case it gets in the eye and causes irritation. Take a dose of aspirin or other analgesic for pain relief. If the eye continues to hurt, apply further cold compresses when required.

Blackouts

Q I black out at the sight of blood and when I am getting an injection. Why?

A Fainting of this sort may be an inconvenience, but usually it is caused by nothing more than having a somewhat oversensitive personality.

Q My father had a blackout recently, and his doctor blamed it on his tight collar. Why would this happen?

A If a collar is too tight or stiffly starched, it may press on a small organ in the neck called the carotid sinus. Heart output is then decreased through a reflex action, thus diminishing the blood supply to the brain. Some people still wear a starched collar, and if they have a sensitive carotid sinus, they may be subject to this kind of fainting. Men who put on weight also often have this problem, which can be relieved quite easily by buying shirts with a larger collar size.

Q I sometimes feel very dizzy when I stand up suddenly. Does this mean that I am having a blackout?

A Unless you actually lose consciousness, you are not having what most people understand to be a blackout. The dizziness is simply the result of a brief drop in the supply of blood to the brain as the heart adjusts to pumping blood "uphill." Most people have experienced this sensation at some time in their lives, and it should be a cause for alarm only if it is repetitive or leads to an actual blackout. However, it is sensible to stand up less abruptly.

Q Should people who tend to have blackouts be allowed to drive a vehicle?

A If the blackouts are recurrent and unpredictable, driving would be hazardous for both the driver and the public. Anyone who is in any doubt about whether or not they should drive should consult their doctor. In general, if a person doubts their safety on the road, they shouldn't drive.

Blackouts range from simple fainting to a loss of consciousness. Usually their cause is not serious.

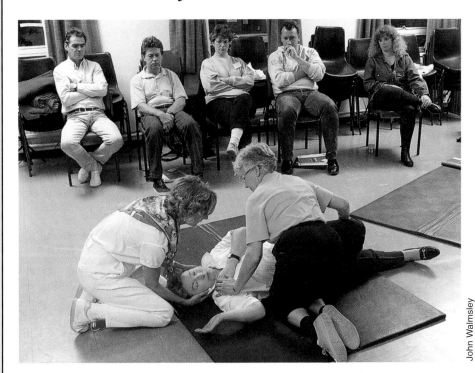

The term *blackout* is most often used to refer to a sudden temporary loss of consciousness called syncope. A faint spell may last for only a few seconds, but more serious blackouts last longer, tend to recur, and are associated with other symptoms that require treatment.

Causes

The brain depends entirely on the bloodstream for a continued supply of essential nutrients, mainly oxygen and glucose. Anything interfering with the amount of blood reaching the brain may result in a blackout. Fainting may occur if a person has been standing for a long time, especially in hot weather, when blood tends to collect in the veins of the lower part of the body. This results in insufficient blood reaching the heart for an adequate flow to be maintained to the brain.

An intensely unpleasant or frightening experience may also lead to fainting (see Fainting): the reflex action of the vagus nerve (the main nerve of the autonomic nervous system) slows the heart, causing the blood flow to the brain to be diminished. Another sort of blackout is the feeling of dizziness or light-headedness when standing up suddenly. This is due to a brief delay in the adjustment of the body to pumping blood to the brain and is no cause for worry.

When a person suffers a blackout, it is vital to arrange the body in a safe recovery position until the doctor arrives. If nasal and mouth secretions are excessive, placing a cushion under the lower half of the body will allow them to drain away safely.

Sometimes, however, the dizziness and light-headedness may occur regularly and result in a complete blackout. This condition, called postural syncope, may indicate some underlying problem of the body's natural mechanisms for maintaining blood pressures. The arteries in the neck that directly supply the brain with blood may be narrowed by atherosclerosis, a disease in which fatty deposits accumulate in the lining of the blood vessels. Degenerative diseases of the spine, such as cervical spondylosis, which affects the neck bones, may also put pressure on these arteries. But patients with this condition faint mainly because they make sudden neck movements that impair blood supply to the brain.

Fainting

Fainting due to a low level of glucose in the blood (hypoglycemia) may occur after several hours without food, especially when coupled with exercise, and in diabetes. Lack of oxygen in the blood (hypoxia) may be due to insufficient

Causes and treatment of blackouts

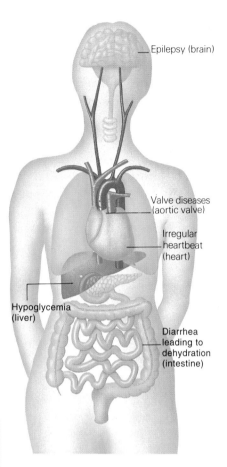

Epilepsy (brain)

Valve diseases (aortic valve)

Irregular heartbeat (heart)

Hypoglycemia (liver)

Diarrhea leading to dehydration (intestine)

Venner Artists

Causes	Treatment
Decreased flow of blood to brain	
Simple fainting (vasovagal syncope)	None needed
Postural syncope (causes temporary unconsciousness)	Treatment of underlying condition
Heart valve disease (may cause fainting on exertion)	Drug treatment Surgery may be considered
Arrhythmias (irregularities of heartbeat)	Pills to regularize heartbeat
Decreased nutrients reaching brain	
Hypoglycemia (low blood sugar)	A lump of sugar or a sweet drink
Anemia resulting in hypoxia (low blood oxygen)	Correction of deficiency (iron, vitamin B_{12}) causing the anemia
Other causes	
Concussion	Requires immediate medical care
Poisons	Requires immediate medical care
Epilepsy	Drug treatment
Hysteria	Attention to emotional disorder underlying the condition

hemoglobin (which carries oxygen in the blood), resulting from lung disease or anemia. Blackouts may also occur due to a temporary upset of normal electrical activity in the brain, and this may be a sign of mild epilepsy (see Epilepsy).

A sharp blow to the head may lead to a blackout or concussion: this is partly due to the temporary high pressures that occur inside the skull because of the blow. Recovery is usually spontaneous (within a few minutes). If prolonged, it may indicate a more serious injury.

Occasionally blackouts may be the result of temporary interruption of blood flow by emboli, small pieces that break off from clots formed in the bloodstream. These may either pass on or break up, but if they do not, they will cause loss of use of the part of the brain concerned.

Symptoms

Aside from loss of consciousness, other symptoms may include nausea, ringing in the ears, and blurring or loss of vision. A cold sweat may appear on the upper lip and the face may turn ashen. The period

of unconsciousness can vary from a few seconds to a few minutes. When loss of consciousness is part of a seizure, there may be a thrashing of limbs and incontinence during the attack. Or there might be nothing more than a flicker of the eyelids. In children, such seizures may pass unnoticed: the child does not fall, but becomes "absent" (motionless and unresponsive) for a few minutes.

Dangers and treatment

There are two kinds of danger: those that arise from the sudden loss of consciousness and those that are caused by an underlying condition.

A blackout when driving may be fatal. Any sudden collapse may cause an injury. While unconscious, there is the danger of breathing being obstructed. If the tongue falls back into the throat, it should be pulled forward. When deeply unconscious, the natural "gag" reflex, which protects the airway, may be missing: if the patient vomits, vomit can block the airway.

Underlying conditions vary in seriousness. Fainting can be a sign of a nervous

personality but recurrent blackouts on standing up may be a warning of a more serious problem. Hypoglycemic blackouts may occur in diabetic patients or may be part of other disorders. Blackouts can also be a symptom of severe anemia.

The most important thing to do if someone has a blackout is to make sure that he or she can breathe properly. Lie the patient on his or her stomach with the head turned to one side, and the arm and leg of that side pulled up. Pulling the chin forward and upward will stop the tongue falling back into the throat. Lift the trunk and legs above head level by placing cushions under the lower half of the body, allowing mouth and nasal secretions to drain out.

A doctor can diagnose the probable cause of blackout and suggest treatment or prevention. An examination will reveal problems such as postural hypotension (a difference in blood pressure when standing and lying). Urine and blood tests can reveal diseases such as diabetes. Where diagnosis is unsure and blackouts persist, referral to a specialist may be necessary.

Bladder and bladder control

The bladder acts as a reservoir for urine. Infection, disease, injury, or stress can cause disorders or loss of control at all stages of life, but most conditions respond well to medical treatment.

Q My urine seems to be a different color on some days. Is this normal?

A Yes. Ordinarily urine is yellow-amber, but it can vary from person to person and will change when certain substances are eaten or drunk. Beets will make the urine redder, as will the dyes in some candies and laxatives made from senna. Some medicines will also discolor urine.

Q I always seem to want to urinate more when the weather is cold. Why is this?

A Bladder function is largely governed by the autonomic nervous system. When you are exposed to the cold, this system acts to retain heat in the body by closing the pores in the skin, which prevents sweating. The liquid that would normally be excreted in this way must then find another way out of the body. The sympathetic nervous system therefore increases the volume of urine produced by the kidneys, and the need to urinate increases.

Q My daughter often holds back from urinating for hours. Will this harm her?

A If signals of a full bladder are habitually ignored, the bladder will eventually stretch, and this may weaken the muscles of its walls and prevent complete emptying. A very full bladder increases the risk of urine being forced back up the ureters toward the kidneys, which may spread infection, if it exists. Perhaps you and your doctor should investigate why she is behaving in this manner.

Q I seem to urinate more frequently than my friends. Do I have a weak bladder?

A Not necessarily. You may have a small bladder, or you may be more attentive to signals from the bladder or less able to override them. People have different metabolic rates; a faster rate creates the need to urinate more frequently. Nervousness also causes more frequent urination.

The urinary bladder is a hollow, thick-walled, muscular organ that lies in the lower part of the pelvic basin between the pubic bones and the rectum. It is a four-sided, funnel-shaped sac resembling an upside-down pyramid. The base of the pyramid provides a surface on which coils of the small intestine, or in women, the uterus, rest.

How the bladder works

The walls of the bladder consist of a number of muscular layers that are capable of stretching while the bladder fills and then contracting to empty it. The kidneys pass an almost continuous trickle of urine down the ureters (the tubes between the kidneys and the bladder). However, rather than the bladder acting like a balloon, with the pressure constantly increasing when it is filled, the muscle fibers of the bladder allow great expansion by adapting to the volume of urine until the bladder is nearly full.

When it begins to resist, the need to pass urine is felt.

The two ureters enter the bladder near the rear edges at the upper surface. One-way valves in the openings where they join the bladder prevent urine from flowing back toward the kidneys if the bladder becomes too full.

Urine is passed out of the body via the urethra, which opens from the lowest point of the bladder. Normally this opening is kept closed by a sphincter, a circular muscle that contracts to seal the passageway. While urinating, this sphincter relaxes at the same time as the muscles of the bladder wall contract to expel the urine.

In women, the urethra is only about 1 in (2.5 cm) long and is not a very efficient barrier against the entry of bacteria from outside, especially if the sphincter is weakened by previous infection, old age, or poor muscle tone. Men are better protected since their urethra has to pass

The urinary systems

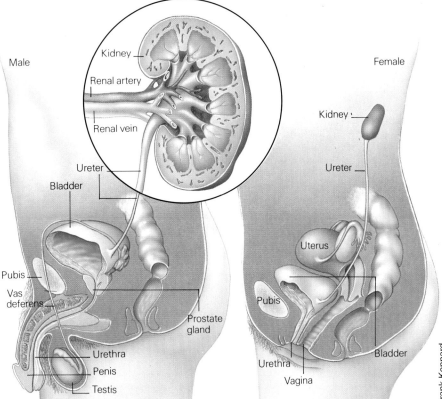

Male — Kidney, Renal artery, Renal vein, Ureter, Bladder, Pubis, Vas deferens, Prostate gland, Urethra, Penis, Testis

Female — Kidney, Ureter, Uterus, Pubis, Urethra, Vagina, Bladder

Frank Kennard

179

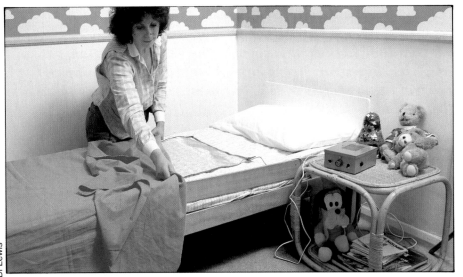

Di Lewis

through the penis and the prostate gland to reach the bladder.

Bladder differences

Although it is commonly thought that women have bigger bladders than men since they need to urinate less frequently, this is not the case. If women are able to postpone urination longer, it is because they have gained greater control over the emptying reflex. By an act of mind over matter, women are able to suppress their body signals more effectively. Bladder capacity can increase to the point where some women only urinate once daily.

Bladder diseases

Cystitis (see Cystitis) is an inflammation of the bladder. It is commonly found in women, because their shorter urethra affords less protection against bacteria. It may be caused by intestinal bacteria that have gotten into the bladder from the anus, from vaginal infections, or from an inflammation originating in an adjacent structure like the kidney. It can occur because of infections contracted through sexual intercourse or childbirth, when there is damage to the urethra after surgery nearby, or when resistance is low.

Symptoms include a constant need to urinate, with scalding pain in the urethra. The urine is either cloudy or may contain pus (pyuria) or blood (hematuria). Pain can also be felt in the pubic area above the bladder, especially before and after urination, and sometimes in the lower abdomen and back.

Cystitis is not usually a serious condition, but there can be psychological distress in addition to discomfort. Treatment is by antibiotics and can last up to two weeks but often the symptoms disappear within the first few days.

An alarm unit can be used to cure bed-wetting habits in children. It is attached to a special bed mat and reacts to wetness by setting off the alarm, thereby waking the child and discouraging bed-wetting.

Other bladder disorders

Kidney stones (calculi) that are too large to pass through the urethra can cause an obstruction and an inability to empty the bladder freely. This condition brings acute distress with colicky pain and requires urgent medical attention. Smaller stones may pass through the urethra, but larger ones may need to be removed by surgery.

Tumors, usually benign, can also be present in the bladder, though sometimes they can become malignant and will require medical attention. The main symptom is the sudden appearance of blood in the urine; there is no pain.

In men, enlargement of the prostate gland in the middle-aged and elderly can obstruct the flow of urine; straining and a decrease in the strength and force of the urinary stream are common symptoms. Others include pain in the prostate region, scalding, painful, and frequent urination, blood or semen in the urine, and difficulties during intercourse and ejaculation. If medical attention is not sought, stones in the bladder or ureter and inflammation of the bladder may develop. A catheter (flexible tube) may have to be passed up the urethra to release the urine that has collected in the bladder.

A fall in the volume of urine passed daily may be due to a narrowing or obstruction of the urethra, an inflammatory condition, drinking less fluid, or spells of hot weather. If obstruction is the cause, the bladder becomes distended and surgery will be needed to relieve the situation.

Any difficulties in urinating or any change in the color of urine due to blood or pus are cause for concern. They may be symptomatic of bladder disease or some disorder elsewhere in the body. Seek medical advice as soon as possible.

Bladder control

Normally the adult bladder will hold up to half a pint (quarter of a liter) of urine before any discomfort is felt, and emptying (micturition) occurs before a full pint has been stored. As the bladder fills, the stretching of the muscle walls passes signals to the spinal cord via nerve endings.

In a small child, this prompts automatic emptying by reflex action. With toilet training, this reflex is gradually suppressed by control from higher centers in the brain. If signs of fullness occur at an inconvenient time, the brain sends orders to the bladder walls to relax and thus allow further filling before the signal is felt again. This process can be repeated several times before the reflex takes over and supersedes voluntary control to prevent damage to the bladder.

Bed-wetting in children

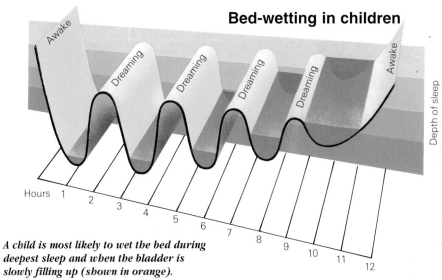

A child is most likely to wet the bed during deepest sleep and when the bladder is slowly filling up (shown in orange).

Bladder problems and their causes

Symptoms	Causes	Action
Scalding pain on urination; cloudy or bloody urine; perhaps pain in lower abdomen and back; no fever	Cystitis (infection of bladder and urethra)	See doctor, who may prescribe antibiotics. If recurrent, drink a lot of fluids; urinate before and after intercourse; avoid panty hose and tight trousers, wear cotton briefs; always wipe genital area from front to back; get enough rest
Inability to empty bladder freely; acute, colicky pain	Stones in urethra	See doctor urgently. Surgical removal of stones possibly needed
Straining and decrease in force of flow of urine in men; blood or semen in urine; difficulties during intercourse or ejaculation.	Enlarged prostate	See doctor. Treatment by catheter if no urine can be passed; probably surgery later
Frequent but scanty urination; urgency; possibly blood in urine	Infection Stones in urethra Tumor	See doctor if condition persists to establish cause
Incontinence	Damage to nerves (stroke, multiple sclerosis, injury to spinal cord, slipped disk) Loss of brain's control over bladder (epilepsy, arteriosclerosis, anxiety) Damage to sphincter of bladder (after removal of womb or prostate)	See doctor to establish cause
Need to get up at night to urinate (nocturia)	Warning of prostate, kidney, or heart trouble	Drink less; urinate before going to bed See a doctor
Bed-wetting (in children over four)	Small bladder capacity from lack of training in retention, or disease Psychological disturbance Chronic bed-wetters in family	See doctor to establish cause. If problem not physical, do not make an issue of it; sensitivity toward child needed. Doctor may prescribe antidepressants

The muscles contract until the bladder is empty. Tensing the abdominal muscles aids this process, although it is normally unnecessary.

Problems of bladder control

Bed-wetting (enuresis) is unavoidable in children up till the age of three or four. However, bed-wetting can also be a problem for older children who have previously been dry, but who have started again after a period of emotional stress, such as the birth of another child in the family. It can also occur in adults as a result of shock or severe emotional problems, or as a symptom of physical illness, such as an obstruction or failure of control by the nervous system, but this is much less common.

Some children stay dry at night earlier than others, and this is probably due to the rate of growth of their bladders, family traits, and home environment. Bed-wetting is more common in boys, but it has nothing to do with intelligence or lack of development.

Over the age of four, confirmed bed-wetting indicates a problem. It may be psychological—resulting from a conflict with parents, or distress at some aspect of home life—or a call for attention. Alternatively there may be a physical reason. Possible underlying causes include chronic urinary infection, injury to the spinal cord after an accident, multiple sclerosis, diabetes, and tumors of the central nervous system.

Congenital abnormalities of the bladder and urethra account for some cases, but an underdeveloped bladder is no cause for alarm. In some families there is a history of chronic bed-wetting, the reason for which has not been determined.

Usually the problem will resolve itself with sensible care by the parents: if bed-wetting becomes an emotionally fraught issue, it will undermine the child's confidence and result in other problems.

Coping with bed-wetting

Avoid giving a child prone to bed-wetting any fluids at bedtime. Take him or her to the bathroom before bed and again before you go to bed. Various methods of toilet training should be used to encourage dryness once the child is old enough to learn. An alarm clock, set at two-hour intervals increasing to six hours, can remind the child when he or she should go to the bathroom. A reward system is sometimes recommended. Otherwise, try a mesh buzzer system—the first few drops of urine set off a buzzer on the bed. But this method may not be successful, because bed-wetting occurs during the deepest sleep, and some children do not awaken. In older children, a doctor may prescribe a drug for a short time to help deal with the problem.

Incontinence

Loss of urine without warning, or an inability to prevent urination, is often present in adults who have had a spinal injury or brain damage or who are very old. Injuries received during childbirth or prostate operations may also cause incontinence, and in women it sometimes occurs as a result of stress and physical exertion.

The inability to control the reflex emptying of the bladder is usually a result of loss of coordination in the nervous system due to injury or disease. The bladder may have to be emptied with a catheter, though sometimes the bladder can be trained to work at planned intervals. Nocturia, the need to get up at night to urinate, may simply be a result of having too much to drink in the evening.

Blindness and Braille

Today many cases of blindness are treatable. But for those who live in darkness or who are partially sighted, the Braille system of reading has improved their lives. Other more modern aids are also now available.

Q I have heard that diabetes can lead to blindness. Could this possibly happen to my sister, who has mild diabetes, and can anything be done in order to prevent it?

A Not all diabetics suffer changes in their eyes, although this is more likely in people who have had diabetes for several years. Only a very small proportion of diabetics actually become blind. Some doctors believe that a patient who keeps a careful watch on his or her sugar levels is far less likely to develop complications, so your sister's best plan is to keep a careful check on this. If eye changes do arise, she must see her doctor at once, and she will probably be sent to an eye specialist.

Q It may sound ridiculous, but I keep getting spots in front of my eyes. Although I am only 23, I can't help worrying that this means that I am going blind. Might this be true?

A You are definitely not alone in your anxiety. This is a common experience that doctors call mucosae volitantes; the little black spots are quite normal and tend to be seen when a person is young and a little anxious. It is not connected with failing vision or blindness in any way at all.

Q My daughter has a bad squint in one eye, and the doctor has suggested that the good eye be covered by a patch to prevent her going blind in the affected eye. Can you explain this treatment?

A Whenever an eye squints, it is out of balance with the other eye. The brain is confronted with two different and confusing images. In children, after a time, one eye takes the lead and the image from the squinting eye is ignored. It never actually becomes blind, but its image is suppressed. If the eye is untreated, it will only be able to distinguish the difference between light and shade. By covering the good eye, the "lazy" eye is forced into use, so the sight is preserved.

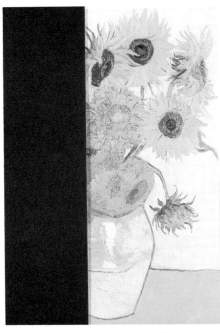

People with partial vision will only be able to see a reduced portion of whatever they are looking at.

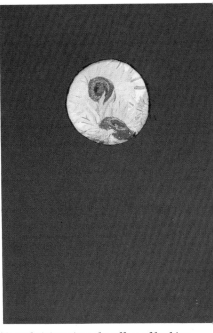

Tunnel vision gives the effect of looking down a tube, and the person only sees a small detail of what is in front of them.

Total blindness, that is, complete loss of vision in both eyes, affects only 5 percent of the people who are called "blind." The majority are, in fact, partially sighted but with deteriorating vision. Such people may only be able to read the number plate of a car at a distance of about three feet (just over a meter), and most are even more handicapped. They can usually see little more than light or shade, or count the number of fingers placed directly in front of them. They live in a dark, blurred, and misty world or have tunnel vision.

Why vision fails

There are many medical causes of blindness or deteriorating vision. The eye is a very complex sense organ, and what a person "sees" outside must be converted first into an image and then into nerve messages, which are interpreted in the brain. Loss of vision can be caused by any interruption of these nerve messages, or it may be the result of an illness, accident, industrial or war injury, or a disease that affects the eye or the nerve pathways within the brain.

Cataracts are one of the principal causes of blindness throughout the world. The clear, transparent lens of the eye becomes opaque, preventing the passage of light and sight gradually fails. The majority of cataracts are caused by the process of aging, but medical conditions or injury to the lens may also cause this problem.

Some children are born with cataracts and in older people, the condition of diabetes is associated with their formation. When the cataract causes a sufficient deterioration of vision so that it must be removed, an operation is performed to remove the damaged lens. The wound is then closed with extremely fine stitches. In most cases, the lens can be replaced with an artificial one; occasionally contact lenses or very thick glasses are prescribed instead.

Blindness in children

Children who are born blind usually have congenital cataracts or have a serious defect of the visual system. Cataracts can be surgically removed, but a condition called nystagmus, which is a fine involuntary tremor of the eye, often occurs and makes focusing extremely difficult. Infections that cause blindness are rare in developed countries, but the most common cause of blindness in the world, trachoma, a virus disease of the eyelids, is still widespread in many underdeveloped tropical regions.

If a pregnant woman contracts rubella (German measles; see Rubella), there is a possibility that her child will be born with cataracts. Similarly, if she should become infested with a tiny parasite of unknown origin, *Toxoplasma gondi*, the child may be born blind.

Young children who are accidentally contaminated with dog excreta while playing outdoors also run a slight risk of contracting the worm parasite, *Toxocara canis*. This can affect the eye and cause chronic inflammation of the retina.

Effects of aging
People who are over 70 may suffer degeneration of the retina, for which there is no cure. The cells of the retina age and die, particularly those in the area called the macula, which is responsible for "fine" vision. Although there is no cure for this condition, its effects can be lessened by magnifying the object.

Magnifying glasses are a practical aid for people with steady hands, but in the aged their use may present a problem.

Closed-circuit television has been used to "blow up" the pages of books or magazines and project them onto a wide screen for easier and closer viewing.

Detached retina
Another common problem in older people is when the retina becomes detached. This happens because the retina is formed from several layers of cells that can be separated from the underlying eyeball. If a tear should also occur, fluid from the eye will leak behind the detachment, making it more difficult to replace.

The first symptom is blindness in the affected eye. This is quite painless, and it seems as if a curtain has descended over the view. Modern techniques have been devised to put the retina back in position, either by surgery or by the use of laser beams. These fuse the retina and eyeball so that they adhere normally, thus saving the person's sight. A detached retina may also happen to younger people after a severe blow to the eye.

Glaucoma
Older people are also prone to a condition called glaucoma (see Glaucoma), when the pressure of the fluid within the eye is raised. The tension within the eyeball produces intense pain, and the delicate nerves transmitting sight become

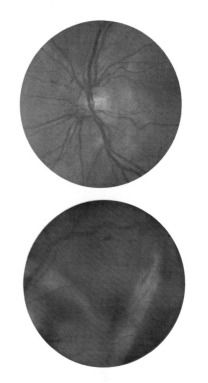

A normal retina (top) contrasted with one damaged by a blow (bottom).

Audiovisual Dept, St Mary's Medical School

compressed and damaged. In acute cases, the rise in pressure happens suddenly, and the eye becomes very painful and red. If this is untreated, vision will be completely and permanently lost.

In chronic glaucoma, the rise in pressure is slow and progressive, so the condition is symptomless. What happens is that the outer boundaries of vision are gradually lost until only tunnel vision remains. This effect can be imagined by looking through a cardboard tube—the vision through the center of the tube is perfect, but anything outside this area is not seen at all. Both surgery and drug treatment can help, but preventive measures are also important. In people over 60, an optometrist should check the pressure within the eye every two years or whenever glasses are changed. Glaucoma can also occur in younger people after an injury or inflammation of the eye.

Other causes of blindness
Any condition that affects the optic nerve or the visual center in the brain can result in blindness. Inflammation of the nerve can be brought about by a viral infection, poisons such as methyl alcohol (hence the expression "blind" drunk), quinine, lead and arsenic, and too much tobacco. When the inflammation is due to the nerve disease disseminated sclerosis, it is often accompanied by a paralysis of the nerves that move the eyeball, which in turn produces double vision.

How the brain enables us to see

The optic nerves carry information from the retinas. At the optic chiasma, information from each eye is transferred to the opposite side of the brain. Depth is analyzed in the lateral geniculate body, and the remaining image is processed in the visual cortexes.

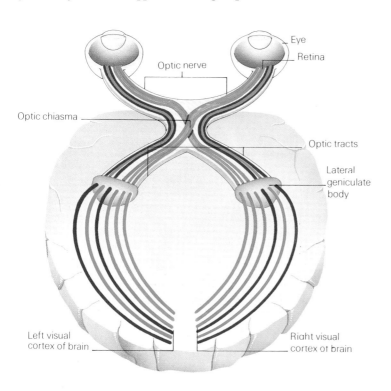

Eye
Retina
Optic nerve
Optic chiasma
Optic tracts
Lateral geniculate body
Left visual cortex of brain
Right visual cortex of brain

Q I have been told that I need to have my cataracts removed next year. I am scared, because when my father had this operation some years ago, he had to lie absolutely still in bed for two weeks. Because he moved when he was told not to, the operation was unsuccessful and he lost the sight in one eye. Can this still happen today?

A You can be totally reassured. These days, thanks to the operating microscope and tiny hair-thin stitches, eye surgery is very different. Healing takes place safely and quickly, so the patient has no need to lie still. In addition, modern local anesthetics are so good that it is not always necessary to have a general anesthetic, and the patient can just be drowsy and comfortable throughout the operation.

Q My 17-year-old son was recently blinded in an accident. Is there any way I can help him to adjust and find possible new careers?

A Helping him to adjust will need all the understanding and love you can give. You can get lots of practical help from your local institution for the blind. As with any normally sighted person, his choice of career will depend on his intellectual or physical capabilities and interests. When all these things have been determined, the many modern aids for the blind mean that your son still has a great deal of choice left open to him.

Q The use of Braille is very widespread these days, but it seems complicated to me. Is it difficult for people to learn?

A Braille is a system that can only be used when both touch and memory are intact. But it is extremely easy to learn and use, especially if the person is blind from childhood. For those with arthritis or poor sensitivity in their fingers, there is the simplified Moon's system, consisting of dots and other characters. Both Braille and Moon enable the blind to read books, periodicals, and sheet music with ease and enjoyment.

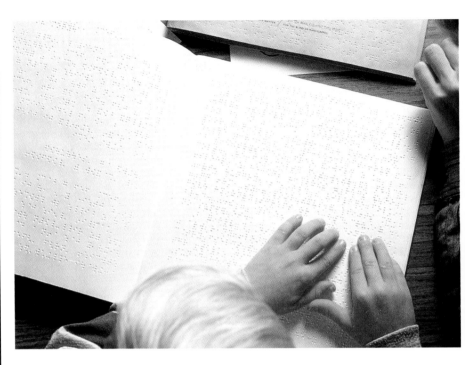

Vision can be partially lost if there is pressure on the optic nerve along its route to the visual center. A tumor, hemorrhage, or dilated blood vessel can produce complicated symptoms that need examining and treatment by a specialist.

Sudden blindness due to a blockage in the blood supply to the retina usually occurs in one eye only. A clot in the artery that supplies the retina will cause instant blindness in the affected eye. It is not curable, but treatment of the medical condition causing it may prevent a similar episode occurring in the remaining "good eye."

A clot in the vein leading from the retina will also produce instant loss of sight, but this may return gradually over several weeks. Subsequent treatment with anticoagulants will be needed to prevent further occurrences.

Diabetes, kidney failure, and extremely high blood pressure are all conditions that can damage the retina, through ruptures of its tiny blood vessels and leakage of protein (exudates). Although there is no definite cure, sight can sometimes be improved by the use of laser beams to seal off the affected areas so that the remainder of the retina can still function.

Retinitis pigmentosa, when patches of pigment form on the light-sensitive retina, is a condition that unfortunately runs in families. As in glaucoma, tunnel vision results. Also, because the periphery (outer area) of the retina is linked with night vision, people with this problem have difficulty seeing in the dark. At the moment, there is no successful treatment and total blindness usually results by the age of 50.

This blind boy has been taught to use the Braille system and is using it to do his math homework.

Living in the dark

Because totally blind people live in complete darkness, they rely on touch, memory, smell, and sound, and over a period of time, these senses heighten considerably. When children are blind from birth, adaptation to this state is part of their development, but those who become blind in later life may be slow to learn.

Some blind people manage to lead fairly independent lives, helped by an understanding partner or with the companionship of a specially trained guide dog—others cannot adapt to their condition and need institutional care.

Most areas have social workers who are trained to identify the needs of the blind and advise on their eligibility for financial assistance and training.

The Braille system

Nearly a hundred years ago, a brilliantly simple idea brought the written word to the blind. This was the Braille system of reading. It was invented by a Frenchman, Louis Braille, who was born in Paris in 1809, the son of a shoemaker. Braille became blind in early childhood as a result of an accident with his father's tools. Despite this, he went on to develop his reading system and also became an excellent musician.

With the Braille method, raised dots are made on paper. The symbols are all variations of a basic six-dot pattern. They are felt with the tips of the fingers, and each group of dots stands for a letter, number or punctuation mark. The reading is done by passing the fingers from right to left.

In Grade 1 Braille, every word is fully spelled out, so reading is slow. In Grade 2 Braille, various contractions and word prefixes speed up the reading. This is the most commonly used version of the system. There is also a Grade 3 Braille for experts, as well as a Braille shorthand.

Braille symbols can be placed on tools and instruments and even on maps and electronic circuits. Writing in Braille is performed by using a punch machine.

One problem is that the dots sometimes become flattened. Recently, plastic dots, which are heat-sealed onto paper, have been used, and these are much longer lasting than the paper symbols.

Electronic aids

Today science is opening up new worlds. Besides television reading aids, talking books and cassette tapes, sonar aids are being developed to help detect objects in a blind person's path.

Helping blind people

Do

- learn the correct way to guide a blind person—for walking, sitting, traveling, etc.

- behave normally when introduced; don't be afraid to say, "Nice to see you."

- say, "Hello," and tell him or her who you are; touch them on the arm

- offer your help in crossing the road

- in your home, show the blind guest around the room, describing the furniture

- describe food that you are offering

- put your cat outside for a while if your blind guest has a guide dog

Don't

- "back" a blind person into a seat— they may end up on someone's lap!

- overdo the sympathy

- say, "Guess who this is."

- try to avoid a blind person in case you are snubbed

- leave cupboards open at head level, put flowers in unstable vases on low tables, leave obstacles such as footstools, toys, etc. on the floor or leave loose floor coverings where a blind person could trip over them

- fill a cup or glass to the brim, especially when serving hot liquids such as tea or coffee

Causes of blindness

Causes	Symptoms	Treatment
Cataract	Gradual onset of misty vision, occasionally double vision	Regular change of eyeglasses while cataract matures. Surgical removal, then lens implant, cataract eyeglasses or contact lenses
Glaucoma (acute)	Painful red eye, persistent headache, often raised blood pressure. Loss of vision	Check on optic pressures every two years or when testing for new eyeglasses. Drugs lower pressure and stop deterioration of vision
(chronic)	Slow, symptomless loss of peripheral vision; tunnel vision	If drug treatment fails, operation to relieve pressure necessary to save sight
Macula degeneration	Mostly affects older people. Both eyes affected, but often one more than the other. Difficulty in reading small print, threading needles, and recognizing faces	No cure. Magnifying glass or closed-circuit television helps to enlarge image so that reading is possible. Telescopic reading glasses help in early stages. Sometimes vitamins and correction of anemia help
Optic neuritis	Sudden loss of vision or blurred vision, great variation of symptoms	If the cause is disseminated sclerosis, treatment is with steroid drugs. If the cause is tobacco poisoning, smoking has to stop
Brain tumor or stroke	Slow or sudden onset, complete loss of part of visual field in both eyes. Objects to the right or left not noticed	Specialist treatment from a neurologist to remove tumor or retrain patient after stroke
Chronic illness—diabetes, kidney failure, high blood pressure	Gradual loss of vision from hemorrhages and leakage of protein over retina	Prompt treatment of the medical condition. Sealing off hemorrhagic areas with laser can help
Retinal artery occlusion (clot in artery) or thrombosis of the retinal vein	Sudden, painless loss of vision in one eye. Vision goes out as if "switched off." In some cases, an accompanying headache	Preventive treatment for any condition that might make it occur in the good eye. Anticoagulant drugs may help the vein thrombosis. In some cases, there is gradual return of sight
Retinitis pigmentosa	Night vision lost initially. Loss of peripheral vision leads to clumsiness. Occurs in families	None found. "Miracle cures" are not likely to bring about anything other than disappointment
Detached retina	Onset in a matter of seconds, like a mist coming over the eye. May be preceded by "flashing lights"	Surgical treatment only. Sealing a tear sometimes possible with laser beam

Blisters

Q I have a huge blister on my heel. Should I pop it?

A Generally it is best to leave blisters as long as possible before popping them because of the risk of infecting the underlying skin. Some blisters (less than 0.75 in or 2 cm across) will be a little more comfortable if the fluid is drained with a sterile pin or needle, but unless these blisters are uncomfortable, they are best left alone, protected by a small bandage. All large blisters require medical attention.

Q My brother is about to start a job on a building site. How can he avoid blistering his hands?

A In the two weeks before he begins work, your brother's skin can be hardened by an application of either very diluted methylated spirit or formalin three times a day. Once he is at work, he should wear well-fitting gloves. When handling tools, the secret is to grip the implement firmly. A loose grip allows more movement between skin and handle, producing more heat and friction, causing a blister.

Q My father, who is 60, keeps developing large blisters on his arms and wherever he scratches himself. Why?

A These blisters are definitely not ordinary friction blisters, but are more likely due to a skin condition called pemphigoid. It is not serious but will require quick attention with steroid drugs to prevent it from spreading. The same symptom in a younger person could herald the beginning of the serious skin disease pemphigus, for which immediate medical attention should be sought.

Q My teenage daughter's new shoes always blister her feet. Can she prevent this?

A Often the cause of blistered feet is shoes that are either poorly fitting or badly designed. Sometimes, however, the shoes merely need to be "broken in."

Blisters can be extremely painful, but if left alone, most will heal by themselves. If one becomes infected or is the symptom of another illness, medical treatment of the blister will be required.

The skin has two layers. The outer one, the epidermis, consists of layers of dead skin cells and contains no nerve cells or blood vessels. The deeper one, the dermis, contains both vessels and nerves. When fluid collects between the two layers, a blister is formed. A small, well-defined buildup of fluid is called a vesicle; larger ones, often up to 3 in (7.5 cm) across, are called bullae.

Causes

Blisters can be caused in a variety of ways. The most common blister is that caused by friction. Rubbing or chafing produces friction and heat, and in response to the heat, a blister is formed. New shoes can chafe areas of tender skin, and walking long distances will often raise blisters.

A person unused to manual labor, who suddenly has to shovel heavy sand, can get blisters within 30 minutes of beginning work. On the other hand, someone accustomed to manual labor, who has

Ray Duns

The blister on this finger was covered by an adhesive bandage to give it protection.

thickened skin, can work for many hours without any trouble at all.

All types of burns, including severe sunburn, can raise blisters. The heat and damage to the deep layer of the skin causes an almost immediate outflow of fluid from the blood capillaries, which then lies in the form of blisters under the skin. Sunburn blisters (see Sunburn) tend to be small and numerous; the skin will start to peel a few days later.

In response to acute inflammation, tiny blisters may sometimes form around the site of an insect bite or a jellyfish sting. In more severe cases, large blisters may form, or they may become infected and fill with pus.

Another common cause of blisters is the inflammation produced by viruses. Chicken pox in children and shingles in adults are caused by the same virus. Shingles blisters are usually confined to one area of the body and may be painful and uncomfortable. Medical attention should be sought, particularly if the patient's eyes or ears are affected.

Chicken pox blisters are far more widespread, covering the trunk and back, and in severe cases, the scalp, the inside of the mouth, ears, and genitals, and they may cause intense itching. When healing, both types of blisters burst: scabs are then formed, which eventually fall off. The virus that causes smallpox, another blister-producing condition, is no longer active in any part of the world.

The herpes simplex virus, which in some people lives within the deep layer of the skin, produces a blister that is called a cold sore. These appear on the lips or side of the mouth after a cold. If

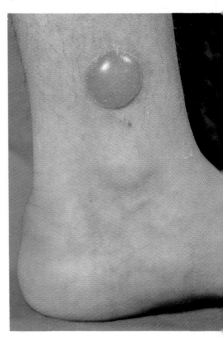

This blister on a woman's leg is the result of an insect bite.

How to treat a blister

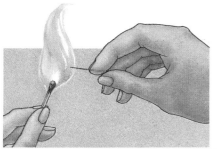

First sterilize a needle to reduce the risk of infection.

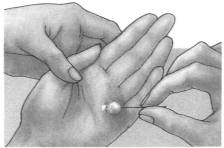

Holding the affected part of the body still, prick the blister.

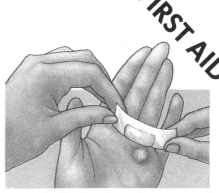

Once the fluid has drained away, cover the blister with a clean dressing.

FIRST AID

Nigel Osborne

the cold is severe or the skin is exposed to excess sunlight, the virus will multiply, and crops of blisters will form.

Bacterial infections can also produce blisters. In impetigo, the bacteria breed quickly in the deep layer of the skin. Small blisters will form, usually on the hands, legs, or face; these soon burst and form crusty, yellow-brown scabs.

In rare cases medical conditions, such as deep vein thrombosis or severe edema caused by heart failure, will produce blistering. More commonly, blisters that result from skin conditions, such as allergic eczema or chemical irritation, will appear without any history of rubbing or burning. Medical treatment is needed.

Two other conditions produce blisters. Pemphigoid causes blistering on the forearms of elderly people, and though the blisters rarely spread or are harmful, they do require some treatment.

Pemphigus, on the other hand, occurs in younger people. It arises because the layers of the skin lose the ability to stay together; the cause of this breakdown of adherence is unknown. Blisters can spread over the whole body, causing severe fluid loss and illness. This condition requires urgent treatment.

Symptoms

The common friction blister causes feelings of heat and pain, and by the time these have been noticed, a blister will have formed. Similarly, in a blister arising from a direct burn, the blister appears a few minutes after the accident.

Blisters from stings and bites appear more slowly and cause itching and swelling of the surrounding skin. Chicken pox begins as small, dark red pimples, which within a few hours turn into blisters that look like droplets of water.

Where there are multiple blisters with no symptoms, the cause is more likely to be eczema. With large blisters, pemphigoid or pemphigus may be the cause, particularly if the blisters arise painlessly, with little or no attendant itching.

Dangers

The common friction blister is rarely dangerous, but in all other types of blister there is a danger of infection. Once the skin of the blister is broken, bacteria can enter and breed, forming pustules, and this will delay healing or spread infection. Where large areas of the skin are blistered, there is also a risk of the body becoming fluid-deficient, causing the patient to become seriously ill.

Treatment

A blood blister should never be burst, and other blisters should be burst only if they are painful or very large. Small blisters are usually reabsorbed, but large blisters generally burst on their own.

To treat a friction blister, for example, on the heel, cool and clean the area. Cover a small blister with an adhesive bandage. If the blister has been caused by new shoes, pad the area with cotton. If there is further friction, release some fluid using a sterile needle. Cover the blister with a bandage and repad the area.

Medical treatment is required for blisters caused by skin inflammations or other illnesses. Antiviral lotions may be of help in virus infections such as shingles. Bacterial infections, such as impetigo, require antibiotic treatment, either applied locally as a cream or taken orally.

Outlook

Provided the friction has ceased, friction blisters will heal within three or four days. The skin will develop a new epidermis, and hard pads may form. Other blisters heal once the underlying cause has been treated, but with chicken pox, new crops of pox may develop while the virus is still alive. Pemphigus is chronic and is controlled by the use of steroid drugs taken only under medical supervision.

How to avoid blisters on feet

Do
- wear well-fitting footwear. Too tight a shoe causes pressure. Too loose a shoe produces friction where the foot slides inside
- wear comfortable, substantial footwear for long-distance walking
- wear additional wool socks in rigid walking boots
- choose soft socks without ridges
- wash and powder feet regularly

Don't
- wear new shoes for the first time on a long walk. Break them in gradually
- choose walking shoes with internal ridges or ankle supports that rub
- walk in sandals with tight, thin straps or flip-flops, where the shoe is held on only by a single strand between the toes
- wear old, hard socks for walking; clean, soft, wool ones are ideal

How to avoid blisters on hands

Do
- wear soft, thick gloves
- change grip, and put a bandage on the hand when blisters appear
- harden up skin with methylated spirit three times a day for three weeks before doing heavy manual work

Don't
- work with rough, abrasive materials, such as bricks, without wearing gloves
- allow caustic substances, such as mortar, to come in contact with hands
- grip tools loosely, as this allows more movement and friction

Blood

Blood is the vital fluid that circulates around the body and maintains life. How is it made up, and what role does each of its elements play?

Blood is essential to body function. It is pumped by the heart around the interior network of arteries and veins from before birth until death, delivering oxygen, food, and other essential substances to the tissues. In return, it extracts carbon dioxide and other waste products that might otherwise poison the system. Blood also helps to destroy disease-producing microorganisms, and through its ability to clot, it acts as an important part of the body's natural defense mechanism.

What the microscope reveals

Blood is not a simple fluid. Its proverbial thickness is due to the presence of millions of cells, whose activities make it as much a body tissue as bone or muscle. It consists of a colorless liquid called plasma, in which float red cells (also called erythrocytes), white cells, or leukocytes, and very small cells called platelets.

To get an idea of the size of a single blood cell, first imagine the size of a micron—one-thousandth of a millimeter. Each red blood cell is a flattened, doughnut-shaped disc with a concave center and a diameter of about eight microns. It is two microns thick at its edge and one micron thick in the center.

Red blood cells

The red blood cells act as transporters, taking oxygen from the lungs to the tissues. Having done this, they do not return empty, but pick up carbon dioxide, a waste product of cell function, and take it back to the lungs, from where it is breathed out. They are able to do this because they contain millions of molecules of a substance called hemoglobin. In the lungs, oxygen combines very quickly with the hemoglobin to give the red cells the bright red color from which their name is derived. Carried in the arteries, this "oxygenated" blood arrives at the tissues. With the help of enzymes in the red cells, carbon dioxide and water, which are other waste products of cell activity, are locked onto the red cells and taken back to the lungs in the veins.

White blood cells

The white cells in the blood are bigger than, and very different from, their red counterparts. Unlike red cells, all white cells do not look alike, and they are capable of moving by using a creeping motion. Involved in the body's defense against disease, white cells are classified into three main groups, which are known technically as polymorphs, lymphocytes, and monocytes.

The polymorphs, which make up 50 to 75 percent of the white cells, are also subdivided into three kinds. Most numerous are those called neutrophils. When the body is invaded by disease-causing bacteria, these go to work. Attracted by chemicals released by the bacteria, they "swim" to the site of infection and start to engulf the bacteria. As they do this, the granules inside the neutrophils begin to make chemicals that destroy the trapped bacteria. The familiar pus that collects at the site of an infection is the result of the

The sample of blood on this slide shows a mixture of red (erythrocytes) and white (leukocytes) cells.

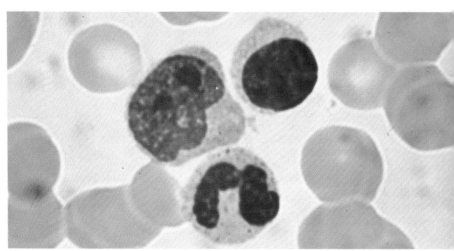

Blood clotting

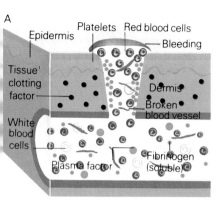

A

Epidermis
Platelets
Red blood cells
Bleeding
Tissue clotting factor
Dermis
Broken blood vessel
White blood cells
Plasma factor
Fibrinogen (soluble)

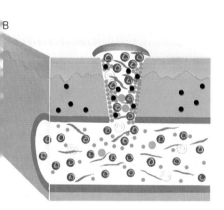

B

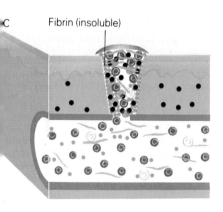

C

Fibrin (insoluble)

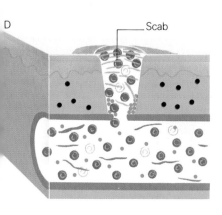

D

Scab

Injured blood vessels bleed and platelets (small, sticky cells in blood) rush to the site to help seal it (A). Tissue-clotting factors are released and plasma factors enter the area (B). The reaction of the platelets, both factors, and other clotting agents convert fibrinogen (a protein) into strands of fibrin that become a jellylike mesh across the break (C). Platelets and blood cells are trapped in this mesh, which now recedes, oozing out serum (liquid blood without clotting factors) that helps form a scab (D). Now bacteria cannot enter the body and cause an infection.

work of the neutrophils and is largely made up of dead white cells.

The second kind of polymorphs are called eosinophils, because their granules become stained pink when blood is mixed with the dye eosin. Composing only 1 to 4 percent of the white cells, eosinophils combat bacterial attack but also have another vital role. When any foreign proteins or antigens get into the blood, substances called antibodies are made to combine with the antigens and neutralize their effects. While this is going on, the chemical histamine is released. The eosinophils lessen the effects of histamine, because if too much is made, the

Where blood cells are made

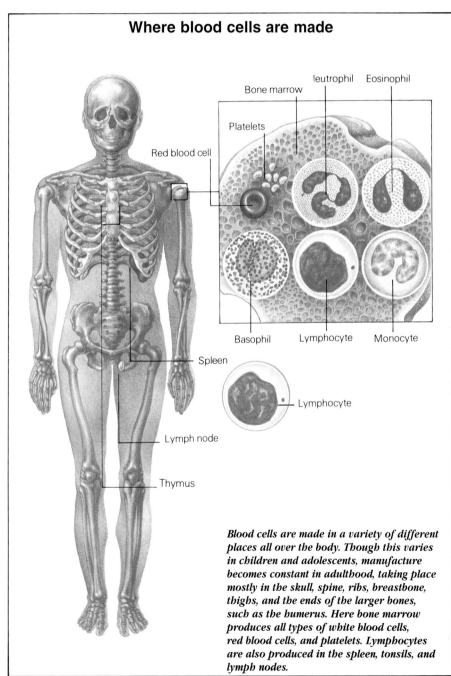

Bone marrow
Ieutrophil
Eosinophil
Platelets
Red blood cell
Basophil
Lymphocyte
Monocyte
Lymphocyte
Spleen
Lymph node
Thymus

Blood cells are made in a variety of different places all over the body. Though this varies in children and adolescents, manufacture becomes constant in adulthood, taking place mostly in the skull, spine, ribs, breastbone, thighs, and the ends of the larger bones, such as the humerus. Here bone marrow produces all types of white blood cells, red blood cells, and platelets. Lymphocytes are also produced in the spleen, tonsils, and lymph nodes.

The functions of red and white blood cells

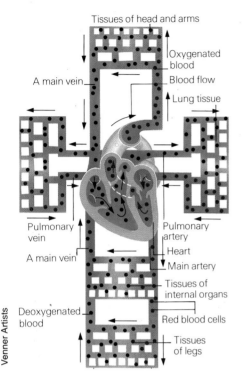

Tissues of head and arms

Oxygenated blood

A main vein

Blood flow

Lung tissue

Pulmonary vein

A main vein

Pulmonary artery

Heart

Main artery

Tissues of internal organs

Deoxygenated blood

Red blood cells

Tissues of legs

Venner Artists

Red cells carry oxygen (oxygenated blood) from lungs to tissues (above left). They then collect carbon dioxide (deoxygenated blood), which is taken to the lungs to be exhaled.

Neutrophil

Nucleus

Neutrophil granule

Digested bacterium

Eosinophil

Cell membrane engulfing bacterium

Antibody-antigen reaction

Nucleus

Histamines

Heparin

Basophil

Nucleus

Antibody

Antitoxin

Lymphocyte

White cells (above right)—neutrophils, eosinophils, basophils, and lymphocytes—fight bacteria, and prevent allergies and clotting of circulating blood.

Contents of one cubic millimeter of blood

Plasma
90–91% water
vitamins
salts
nutrients
hormones
urea

55 %

platelets 250,000
white cells 10,000

red cells
5,000,000

45 %

result can be an allergic reaction. Once the antibodies and antigens have combined, the eosinophils remove the chemical remains.

The third type of polymorphs are the basophils. Although basophils make up

less than one percent of all white cells, they are essential to life because their granules make and release heparin, which works to stop the blood from clotting inside the vessels.

Natural immunity

Making up about 25 percent of the blood's white cells are the lymphocytes, which all have dense, spherical nuclei (centers). Lymphocytes (see Lymphocytes) also play a vital role, giving the body its natural immunity to disease.

They do this in two ways. The "B" lymphocytes, made in the lymph nodes and spleen, produce antibodies to counteract the damaging effects of bacteria and their toxins (poisons). The antibodies combine with these foreign substances to neutralize and make them harmless.

The "T" lymphocytes, made in the thymus, kill foreign tissue elements and infectious organisms, and may also protect the body against its own cells when they undergo malignant change. The T lymphocytes also secrete chemicals that help B cells function.

Last of the white cells are the monocytes, which form up to 8 percent of the white cells. The largest monocytes

contain large nuclei that engulf bacteria and remove the debris of cell remains, resulting from bacterial attack.

The millions of minute platelets in the blood are similar to the red cells in having no nuclei. The platelets all have sticky surfaces, and this is a clue to their function. If the minute blood vessels called capillaries (see Capillaries) are damaged, chemicals are released that make the platelets stick to the broken ends and plug them to stop the bleeding. The platelets also help trigger blood clotting.

The clotting process

The ability of the blood to clot, or coagulate, and so prevent bleeding to death if a blood vessel is severed, comes from the combined action of the platelets and a dozen biochemical substances called clotting factors. Among these is the important substance called prothrombin. The factors are found in the fluid part of the blood—the plasma—and are called plasma factors. Defects of the clotting process are of two kinds—failure of clots to form and thrombosis, in which blood clots form in the vessels.

Plasma

Although about 90 percent of it is water, plasma (see Plasma) is packed full of vital chemicals that it carries around the body. Among these are vitamins, minerals, sugars, fats, and proteins—in fact, all the constituents needed for cell function and renewal. Just as the blood cells carry away cell waste, so, too, does the plasma. The most concentrated chemical refuse in the plasma is urea, which is ferried to the kidneys for excretion in the urine.

Manufacture of red blood cells

The production of red blood cells begins in the first few weeks after conception, and for the first three months, manufacture takes place in the liver. Only after six months of fetal development is production transferred to the bone marrow, where it continues for the rest of life. Until adolescence, the marrow in all the bones makes red blood cells, but after the age of 20, red cell production is confined to the spine, ribs, and breastbone.

Red blood cells begin their life as irregular, roundish cells called hemocytoblasts, with huge nuclei. These cells then go through a rapid series of divisions, during which the nucleus becomes progressively smaller and then is lost altogether.

In their travels around the bloodstream, the red cells are subjected to enormous wear and tear and so need constant renewal. Each red cell has an average life of 120 days. After this, cells made in the bone marrow and spleen attack those blood cells that are worn

Causes and treatment of diseases affecting blood clotting

Disease	Underlying causes	Treatment
Hepatitis, cirrhosis, and other liver disorders	Deficiency of prothrombin and other clotting factors of the plasma, made in the liver	Rest, nourishing diet
Gallstones or other interference with bile production or the release of bile	Vitamin K made in the intestine by bacteria is poorly absorbed into the blood in the absence of bile. Lack of vitamin K leads to low prothrombin production	Vitamin K injections, treatment of underlying cause
Hemophilia	Deficiency of clotting factors. Found only in males, the condition is inherited. Women can be carriers but do not suffer from it	Rest in bed after any injury, blood transfusion, Factor VIII. Preparation containing thrombin applied to wounds
Purpura—bleeding into the skin or joints that may cause tiny bruises or bleeding spots on the body	Low numbers of platelets. Many causes, including side effects of drugs, viral diseases, bone marrow disease. Or platelet numbers normal but their function impaired. Causes include scurvy, allergies, or fragile capillaries. Caused by allergies, prolonged cortisone treatment, or deterioration of capillaries in old age	Treatment of underlying cause. Blood transfusions and extra iron may be needed

White blood cell disorders

Disease	Types of disorder	Causes
Leukocytosis	Overproduction of white cells, particularly neutrophils	Infections, particularly glandular fever. Aftereffect of heart attacks
Eosinophilia	Too many eosinophils (type of white blood cell)	Allergies such as asthma and hay fever. Worm infections
Leukopenia	Too few white cells, particularly all types of polymorphs	Tuberculosis, typhoid, and some viral infections. Side effects of certain drugs including chloramphenicol, sulfonamides. Side effect of radiotherapy
Leukemia	Too many white cells, but extra cells abnormal	Cancer of the bone marrow or lymphatic system. Some types may be caused by viruses

out. Some of the chemical remains are immediately returned to the plasma for reuse, while others, like hemoglobin, are sent to the liver for further destruction.

The body has a remarkable ability to control the number of circulating red cells, which it does according to its needs. If a lot of blood is lost, or parts of the bone marrow are destroyed, or the amount of oxygen reaching the tissues is decreased—due to heart failure or high altitude, for example—the bone marrow immediately begins to increase red blood cell production. Even strenuous daily exercise (see Exercise) stimulates extra red cell output, because the body then has a regular need for more oxygen.

Manufacture of white blood cells
The bone marrow is also the site of some white blood cell manufacture. All three types of polymorphs are made here from cells called myelocytes, again by a series of divisions. The average polymorph lives only 12 hours, and only two or three hours when the cells are involved in fighting bacterial invasion. In such circumstances, the output of all white cells is increased to meet the body's demands. The lymphocytes, which live an average of 200 days, are made in the spleen, and in areas such as the tonsils and the lymph glands scattered throughout the body. Both monocytes and platelets are made in the bone marrow. The exact length of

monocyte life is a mystery, for they seem to spend part of their time in the tissues and part in the plasma, but the body manages to replace all its millions of platelets on average about once every four days.

Although bleeding should always be taken seriously, the body's inborn survival mechanisms insure that a person can lose a quarter of his or her blood without suffering long-term ill effects, even if a blood transfusion is not given. Because blood is the supply line to and from the tissues, disorders and diseases show up via alterations in the blood. Apart from being a reflection of the body's state of health, the blood itself can be the site of a range of disorders, each requiring treatment.

Blood donor

Q I would like to give blood but I'm frightened it will hurt. Can you reassure me?

A Yes. Your thumb is first pricked to obtain a drop of blood for the hemoglobin test. Then, before the needle is put into your arm for the blood donation, you are given a local anesthetic that numbs the skin. You will feel a gentle pumping sensation as your blood is drawn—and that is all.

Q I have a job that involves a lot of heavy lifting. Will giving blood make me too weak to work?

A No. In a recent experiment, a group of doctors were blindfolded. Half had some blood taken, and the other half just had the needle slipped under the skin but no blood taken. When all the donations were finished, the needles were taken out and the blindfolds removed. The donors then did a series of exercises and tests. There was no difference in the performance of the two groups.

Q I have a common blood group (type). Is my blood of any use?

A Definitely. Most of the people who require blood transfusions will have common blood groups, so your blood is just as valuable as blood from a person who has a rare group.

Q My sister has just recovered from hepatitis. Will this prevent her from becoming a blood donor?

A This depends on the type of hepatitis. If she has had hepatitis A, there is no obstacle to giving blood after convalescence is complete. If the disease was hepatitis B and there is persistent viral antigen in her blood, your sister is permanently barred from donating. In addition, if she has a history of hepatitis, and blood studies show no proof of its being A or B, but certain liver function tests are abnormal, again there is a permanent ban on your sister donating blood.

Every minute of every day, someone, somewhere requires a blood transfusion. It only takes a few minutes to donate a pint of blood, and this painless procedure could save a life.

Anyone between the ages of 18 and 65 who is in good health can donate blood. People with heart conditions, high blood pressure, kidney, thyroid, or blood disease, or who have had tuberculosis, syphilis, or certain cancers are barred. Pregnant women, people who have recently had an operation or a tooth extracted, or who are anemic, must wait a certain period of time before they can donate. If a person's occupation or hobbies are particularly active or hazardous, they will only be accepted if at least 12 hours have elapsed, during which their blood will have regained its strength.

Initial checks

At the donation clinic, a potential donor will be given a sheet that lists the conditions that may prevent a person from giving blood. The first section of questions is designed to protect the donor: he or she may be someone who could be harmed by a mild lowering of blood pressure, for example. The second section is aimed at protecting the person to whom blood might be given. Some bacteria and viruses that cause disease can be carried in the bloodstream. If a donor is suffering from one of these diseases, is incubating it, or has recently been immunized against it, the organisms would be transferred into the recipient, so the donor cannot give blood.

The donor will also be checked for anemia. A doctor or nurse pricks the thumb and takes one drop of blood, which is put into a bottle of copper sulfate solution. If the drop sinks within 15 seconds, the donor is not anemic and is allowed to give blood. If the drop does not sink within the required time, a sample of blood will be taken for further tests, and the donor will be referred to his or her own doctor for treatment.

A donor will be asked his or her name, age, and address, so that their donation can be identified and a record sent to them. Then he or she will lie down on a bed. The donor attendant will roll up a sleeve and put a blood pressure cuff on the upper arm. This is pumped up to a pressure that allows blood to flow into the arm, but prevents it from returning.

What happens next

The doctor who is going to take the blood sterilizes the skin in the crook of the arm by rubbing it with alcohol. He or she then gives a small injection of local anesthetic above the vein from which the donation will be taken. This stings momentarily, but within seconds the skin is numbed. The doctor then puts a needle into the selected vein.

The donor's blood flows into the blood collection bag, which is attached to the needle. The bag, which is hung on a special balance that cuts off the blood flow to the bag once the required amount of

The doctor checks the pack in which the blood will be collected. The donor on the right is resting before going home.

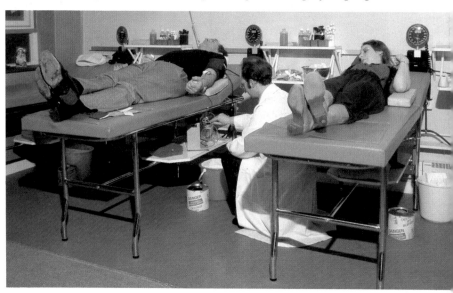

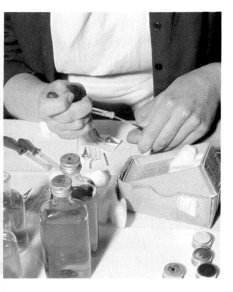

The donor is tested for anemia before being allowed to give blood.

blood has been taken, contains a colorless fluid. This is a mixture of anticoagulant, to prevent the blood from clotting, and dextrose, a sugar, to nourish the blood cells while they are being stored.

After about 10 minutes, the donation will be complete. The amount of blood taken, 0.75 pint (426 ml) represents about one-twelfth of a person's circulating blood. The volume is made up from the extracellular fluid within 20 minutes, but until this happens, there is a slight chance of fainting. To prevent this, a donor is asked to remain on the bed while having a drink and eating a cracker.

The other components of the blood take longer to replace: the plasma content takes 24 hours, but the red cells take up to six weeks. A blood donor will not be allowed to give another donation for at least another three months.

The donated blood is then sent to the central processing laboratory, where it is blood-grouped and screened for hepatitis, syphilis, and atypical antibodies.

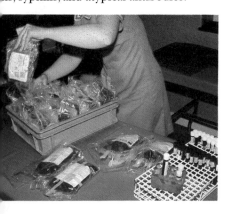

An assistant collects the carefully labeled donations for the laboratory.

Reasons for delaying blood donorship

Disease	Person who suffered from disease must delay	Person in contact must delay
Glandular fever	1 year	3 months
Jaundice or hepatitis	See question and answer section opposite	
Brucellosis (undulant fever)	Permanent ban	
Malaria	3 years since last attack	12 weeks after leaving malarious area
Other tropical diseases	Varying periods	—
Minor illnesses (flu, sore throat, boil)	One week after cleared up	—
Infectious fevers (measles)	See text	Incubation period
AIDS	Permanent ban	Pending HIV testing

Other reasons for delay

Reason	Waiting period
Tattooing, acupuncture, ear piercing	6 months
Receiving a blood transfusion	6 months
Immunization or vaccination:	
Live vaccine (e.g., polio)	2 weeks
Dead vaccine (e.g., cholera)	1 day
Treatment with certain drugs (e.g., antibiotics or antihistamines)	Duration of course of treatment

Note: Being on the contraceptive pill does not prevent you from being a blood donor.

Uses of donated blood

Donated blood is not only used to replace blood lost, for example, through an accident. Some people have greatly lowered resistance to infection. This may be an unavoidable side effect of giving a patient a bone marrow transplant, or treating leukemia or other cancers, or a child born with very little natural immunity to disease. Such people are at great risk from what the normal person would consider mild to moderate infections such as a bout of cold sores or the measles. If such a person is exposed to one of these diseases, his or her immunity can be boosted by an injection of antibodies against that disease. Another use of such antibodies is to protect the fetuses of pregnant women who have been exposed to rubella (German measles).

These antibodies are obtained from blood donors who have recovered from the disease in the last three months. Common antibodies obtained are mumps, chicken pox, measles, rubella, and cold sores. Other antibodies collected include tetanus and some rare tropical diseases.

Blood-grouping

Reagents, substances used to cause a reaction so that patients' blood groups can be identified, are mainly obtained from blood donors who have antibodies that will react against a particular blood group, showing that it is incompatible with a certain type of blood. Antibodies, both for reagents and boosting immunity, are usually collected by plasmapheresis, a process whereby the plasma (the colorless fluid in which the blood cells float) is removed.

In an emergency, group O Rhesus-negative blood can be given to almost anyone. For this reason, people with this blood group are known as universal donors. But with modern, rapid techniques of cross-matching, this practice is becoming less common.

Blood groups

Q I know that Rhesus-negative blood is quite rare. What are the most common groups?

A You are right in thinking that Rh-negative (Rhesus-negative) is fairly rare—only 15 percent of the population are without the Rhesus factor. A positive and O positive are the most common groups, and AB negative—shared by a mere 0.45 percent of the population, or about one in 200—is by far the rarest.

Q I had a short-lived affair a few months ago but then split with my lover and returned to my husband. I am now pregnant and my husband does not believe that it is his child. I am sure that it is because of the timing. Is it true that a blood test can reveal who the real father of a child is?

A Blood tests cannot prove that a man is definitely the father, but they can prove that someone is not related to the child. It is impossible to predict with 100 percent certainty what characteristics a child will inherit from the parents. But a child who is Group B, for example, will not have two parents whose blood is either Group A or O.

Q I have Rh-negative blood. What would happen if I was given a transfusion of Rh-positive blood, say after an accident?

A You could get away with such a transfusion—but only once. After the first transfusion, the body would form antibodies to the Rhesus blood cells, but not quickly enough to cause immediate problems. However, those antibodies would stay in your circulation permanently and would react very quickly indeed to a further Rh-positive transfusion.

The antibodies would destroy the red cells in the new blood and clog up your blood vessels and kidneys. The kidneys are the body's principal filtering system, and if prompt action were not taken, such as putting you on a kidney machine, the situation could be fatal. This is why doctors routinely test patients before giving them any kind of transfusion. So you do not need to worry about this happening.

For centuries people assumed that we all had identical blood. Now our knowledge of the different blood groups enables lives to be saved daily.

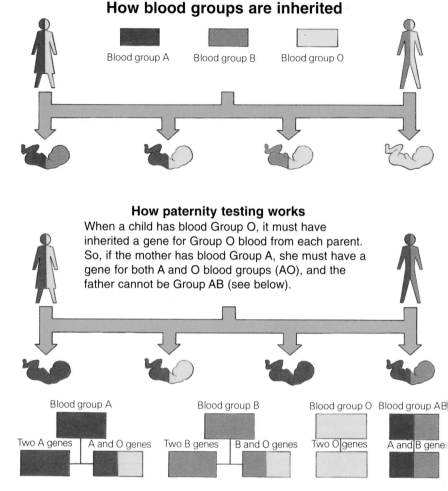

How blood groups are inherited

Blood group A Blood group B Blood group O

How paternity testing works

When a child has blood Group O, it must have inherited a gene for Group O blood from each parent. So, if the mother has blood Group A, she must have a gene for both A and O blood groups (AO), and the father cannot be Group AB (see below).

Blood group A — Two A genes — A and O genes

Blood group B — Two B genes — B and O genes

Blood group O — Two O genes

Blood group AB — A and B genes

The major blood groups were first identified in the 1930s by Viennese doctor Karl Landsteiner. He experimented by mixing blood from a variety of donors and found that only some people's blood could be mixed satisfactorily. He also discovered that, more often than not, mixing blood from different donors would result in massive damage to the oxygen-carrying red blood cells.

Landsteiner identified four blood groups that are now known as A, B, AB, and O. What differentiates the groups is the presence or absence of protein coats on the red cells and of antibodies (which are part of the body's defense system) in the plasma (see Plasma), the colorless fluid part of the blood.

These proteins act rather like a badge or coat of arms: they enable cells to "see" or judge whether other cells belong to the same group as they do or whether they are potentially dangerous outsiders.

Blood tests are often used in paternity cases. But a test will only show that a child is not related to the father; it cannot be used to give positive proof of identity of fatherhood.

If a cell wears a different protein from that of the native cells, it will be attacked and neutralized by the antibodies in the plasma. Group A and Group B red cells each have their own distinguishing protein on their surface.

Compatible groups

People with Group O are called universal donors. Because their blood contains neither distinguishing proteins nor aggressive antibodies, it will be accepted by everyone.

Group AB people are called universal recipients, because they have no antibodies to destroy alien red cells. But although it may be relatively safe to mix blood groups under these circumstances, it is not done in practice. It is always safest to transfuse blood of exactly the same group.

If someone is given a transfusion of the wrong kind of blood, the antibodies in their own blood will attack the red cells in the transfused blood, and the antibodies in the transfused blood will attack the patient's own red cells.

When an antibody attacks a red cell, they both clump together in a sticky mess that clogs up the blood vessels and kidneys. A small transfusion would therefore cause jaundice and fever, while a larger one might block the flow of healthy blood to major organs and eventually lead to the death of the patient. The technical term used for this type of clumping is *agglutination*.

Heredity

A person's blood is determined by heredity (see Heredity). Broadly speaking, if parents have the same blood group as each other, their child will have the same group, too. If one is A (or B) and the other O, the child will be A (or B). If one is A and the other B, the child will be AB.

If it were as simple as this, however, Group O would have disappeared by now, but it is actually the most common group in the world. It survives because anyone with a Group O parent retains what is called a recessive gene; if two people with this recessive gene have a child, his or her blood type is as likely to revert to Group O as it is to follow the pattern described above.

How the Rhesus factor can affect a baby

First pregnancy

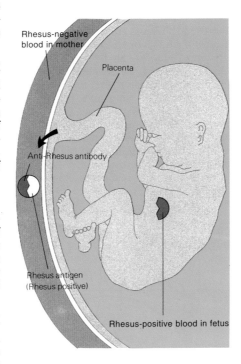

Second pregnancy

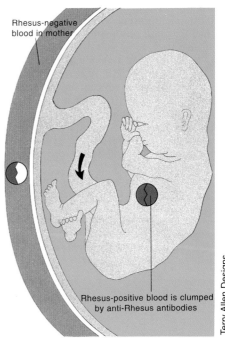

Terry Allen Designs

If the blood from a Rh-negative mother and a Rh-positive baby mixes accidentally during labor, the mother will produce anti-Rh antibodies, but too late to affect a first baby.

If the bloods mix during a second labor, the baby's blood will coagulate, because the mother now has anti-Rh antibodies in her blood as a result of the first baby.

The connection between blood groups and disease

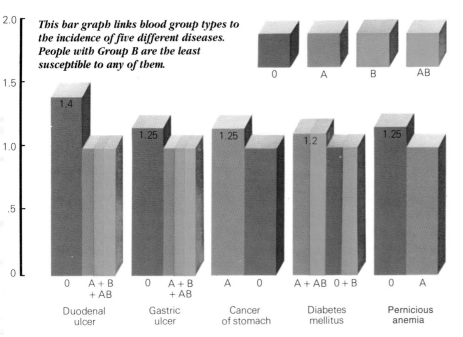

This bar graph links blood group types to the incidence of five different diseases. People with Group B are the least susceptible to any of them.

Certain blood groups are known to be more susceptible than others to particular diseases. For instance, people with Group O blood are more likely to develop duodenal ulcers, gastric ulcers, and pernicious anemia. Group A has a higher incidence of stomach cancer, and Group A and Group AB are more prone to diabetes.

The Rhesus factor

Another very important aspect of blood grouping is the Rhesus factor (see Rhesus Factor), a protein first found in the blood of Rhesus monkeys. Eighty-five percent of white people are Rh-positive, which means that they have the Rhesus factor. It was the discovery of this factor, which can be present in blood of any group, that eventually led to an explanation for what was once quite a common and very dangerous, even fatal, kind of anemia found in newborn children.

Researchers found that these children invariably had a father who was Rh-positive and a mother who was Rh-negative. The strange thing they discovered about this unpleasant condition was that it only affected the mother's second or subsequent children, never the firstborn.

The trouble arises when the Rh-negative mother is carrying an unborn baby with Rh-positive blood. During labor a certain amount of the baby's blood always gets into the mother's bloodstream. The Rh factor is "seen" by the mother's immune system as a foreign invader, and it produces antibodies against it.

There is some transfer of blood from mother to baby and vice versa through the placenta throughout the pregnancy, but it is mostly in labor that the baby is exposed to the mother's blood. However, there is not enough time for the mother's antibodies to build up and get into the baby's bloodstream during the labor of this first pregnancy.

But during subsequent pregnancies, the antibodies that have formed do filter through into the baby, where they start destroying its Rh-positive cells. It can be compared to the progress of an allergy; no symptoms are produced by a first exposure, but subsequent contacts with the offending substance will produce some kind of reaction.

This condition affects one child in 500 and used to lead to stillbirth, severe jaundice, and anemia or serious heart or brain damage. Today it can be prevented by giving the mother an injection of Rh antibodies shortly after the first delivery. These antibodies mop up any of the baby's blood cells that may be floating around in the mother's bloodstream and are themselves consumed before her immune system has had time to produce its own permanent antibodies. So if the woman has another Rh-positive baby, it will face no greater risk than the firstborn baby.

Other ways of grouping blood

In addition to the A, B, AB, and O groups and the Rhesus factor, there are more than a dozen other systems of grouping

How the different blood groups are identified

Whenever red cells from Group A blood encounter the anti-A antibody found in Group B blood, they will stick together (agglutinate). Similarly, if Group B red cells meet the anti-B antibody found in Group A blood, they will agglutinate. Group AB blood cells can be agglutinated by exposing them to either of these antibodies. But Group O cells will remain unharmed by either antibody. The test is carried out by mixing one drop of blood on a glass slide with a preparation containing anti-A serum and another drop of blood with anti-B serum. The analyst then looks at the samples through the microscope to see if they agglutinate.

blood, all of which rely on identifying some kind of distinguishing protein in the blood cells. Two such blood types, called M and N, were also identified by Landsteiner.

For the practicing doctor worried about blood transfusions or the health of individual babies, these other groups are not of any great practical importance. Their principal uses are in the study of heredity and in paternity tests, and they have little significance for health care on a daily basis.

Some hematologists (doctors who are blood specialists) now have such sophisticated techniques that many experts believe that blood grouping will soon prove to be as positive a method of identifying individuals as fingerprinting is known to be.

Ethnic blood groups

There is a definite difference in the percentage of different blood groups in the various ethnic populations throughout the world. In the UK, for example, more people have Group O blood than any other single group; people with Group B blood are a small minority. In India and China, on the other hand, the picture is reversed. In these countries, the largest number of people have Group B blood.

In the US, among the white population, 45 percent are Group A, 43 percent are Group O, 8 percent are Group B, and 4 percent are Group AB. Among African Americans, 29 percent are Group A, 50 percent are Group O, 17 percent are group B, and 4 percent are Group AB. Among Asians in the US, 35 percent are group A, 30 percent are group O, 23 percent are Group B, and 12 percent are Group AB.

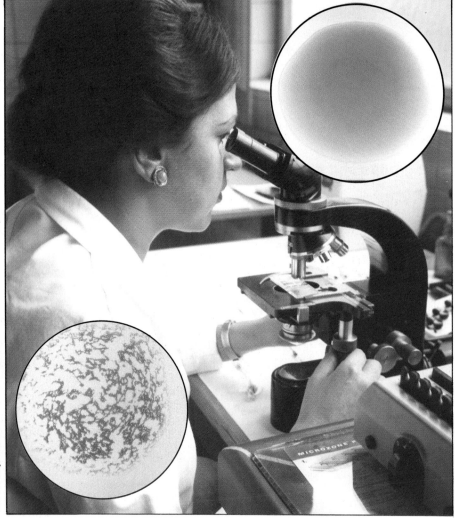

Group A blood (below right) is identified in a laboratory. It has coagulated (below left) after Group B blood, containing anti-A antibodies, has been added.

Blood poisoning

Q My husband works as a mailman, and while he was making deliveries recently, he was bitten by a dog. He checked and found that the animal's rabies vaccine is valid, but I am still worried. Can he get blood poisoning from this?

A He could. A bite can cause an infected wound and can introduce bacteria that cause cellulitis, tetanus that causes toxemia, or an abscess that may break down to cause septicemia. However, dog bites seldom become infected, and blood poisoning is therefore very unlikely. Check that your husband's immunizations are up-to-date, and if the site of the wound forms an abscess or becomes red and painful, he must consult his doctor immediately.

Q Two days ago I cut my finger. But now I am worried because it is discharging pus and is very painful. There is also a red swelling that seems to be spreading up my arm. What can I do about it?

A See your doctor, who will probably prescribe penicillin. This sounds like a clear case of a spreading infection, which needs treatment with antibiotics as soon as possible.

Q The symptoms usually given for both blood poisoning and general viral infections like flu, for instance, seem to me to be very similar. How will I be able to tell the difference between them?

A It is true that it is hard to tell the difference between septicemia or toxemia and a viral infection, because the symptoms—fever, sweating, lethargy, nausea, and loss of appetite—are so similar. But viral infections are usually less severe than those caused by bacteria. With blood poisoning, there will also be signs of the source of the infection (for example, a skin wound). A diagnosis is made by special tests that culture the bacteria from the blood in order to identify the culprit causing the infection. The correct form of treatment can then be prescribed.

Blood poisoning is a bacterial infection that can occur in any part of the body. Proper treatment is essential.

Blood poisoning can occur through a dirty wound becoming infected, the breaking down of an abscess so that bacteria are released into the bloodstream, or an infection in the throat, the lungs, the digestive system, or the urinary tract.

Types

There are two main types of blood poisoning, the most common of which is called septicemia. It is not a localized infection and will spread throughout the body if it is not controlled. The bacteria (see Bacteria) that cause septicemia can enter the blood in a number of ways such as an open wound, a tooth extraction, or infected internal bruising.

Normally the white blood cells will cope by mopping up the bacteria, but if they increase to such a number that the body's natural defenses are overwhelmed, septicemia may result.

The symptoms of septicemia include fever, shock, and prostration, together with a sudden lowering of blood pressure. A patient will feel extremely ill and may lapse into a coma. Death can follow.

Sometimes the body may successfully confine an infection, but this will not stop the bacteria from releasing chemical poisons called toxins into the bloodstream. These can cause a condition called toxemia.

There are two types of toxins. One is made by the bacteria and then excreted, causing separate side effects from those of the original infection. These toxins produce specific symptoms such as the paralysis caused by tetanus (see Tetanus). Second, toxins may be formed naturally inside the bacterial cells, which are then released into the bloodstream after the destruction of the bacteria by either white cells or antibiotics.

A patient with toxemia will feel sick and feverish. He or she will often complain about unpleasant aftereffects if taking antibiotics, but these are caused by the release of the toxins rather than the drugs themselves. Some bacteria can break down the tissues beneath the skin, enabling bacteria to spread under the surface. This is called cellulitis, and it appears as a painful, spreading red halo around an infected wound or abscess.

Treatment

Antibiotics are usually effective in quelling bacterial infections. Preventive medicine is practiced wherever possible, and immunization against tetanus and diphtheria is offered to every infant.

Tattooing is sometimes carried out in an unhygienic manner, and dirty needles may cause blood poisoning.

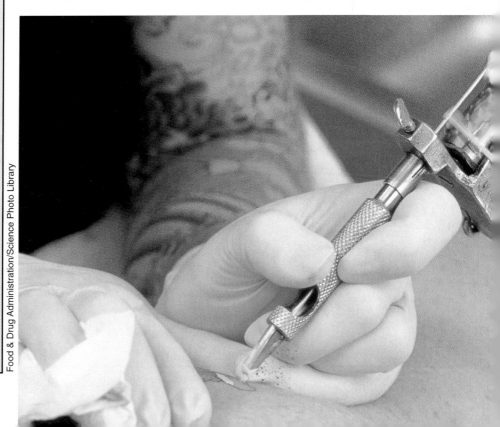

Food & Drug Administration/Science Photo Library

Blood pressure

Q My doctor says I must avoid stress. But how can I do this in my job, which is very tiring and stressful?

A There is a growing volume of evidence that stress can lead to high blood pressure and that avoiding stress will improve blood pressure, even though this is hard to prove in absolute terms. It is therefore reasonable that your doctor should ask you to look at the stresses in your life, because their identification might go a long way toward reducing their effect.

Have you thought about trying one of the techniques that will teach you how to relax? Yoga and breathing exercises, for example, could be very useful this way.

Q I am being given drugs for high blood pressure, but I have read somewhere that these can lead to changes in personality. Is this true?

A Partly. There is no doubt that some of the older drugs can affect mood and can cause depression. For this reason they are now being replaced by others that have reduced side effects. The beta-blocking types of drugs, which block the effects of adrenaline in the body, may affect mood. Some patients fear they will cause them to lose their drive and initiative, but this is not usually the case. The beta-blockers simply reduce the excessive wear on the heart and circulation; they are certainly not depressants. If you experience problems with the drugs you are taking, talk to your doctor about the matter.

Q My doctor has just told me my blood pressure is slightly up. Will this affect my life insurance policy?

A Yes, it will. It was the statistics provided by insurance companies that highlighted the major contribution blood pressure makes to overall mortality in society. Therefore they take keen interest in the results of medical examinations, and trying to cover it up could just make things worse. Own up and pay up—and then get the problem under control.

Blood pressure problems affect many people and are a major cause of ill health. But regular checkups can detect warning signs, and treatment does not usually interfere with a person's normal life.

When blood pressure is raised, a person is said to have high blood pressure, or hypertension, and if this is not treated, the chances of disease—or even death—are increased. In fact, the major causes of death in the Western world today are diseases of the heart and blood vessels. Blood pressure is therefore not just a symptom but an urgent warning signal.

Causes

The trouble starts within the arteries (the thick-walled vessels that carry blood from the heart to the tissues of the body). The blood is driven by the main pumping chamber of the heart, the left ventricle, and a great deal of force is required to send the blood out of the heart and into the arteries, through the tissues, and then back into the heart again to be redelivered to the arteries. Therefore even under ideal conditions, the walls of the arteries are continually under considerable stress.

The level of arterial pressure is of great importance. If the pressure within the system is raised for any reason—a condition called hypertension—this stress is increased and paves the way for the development of arteriosclerosis, a narrowing of the arteries due to the degeneration of the middle coat of the artery walls. The heart and the arteries can be severely strained and damaged by the blood pounding through with a very unnatural force.

On the other hand, seriously low blood pressure, called hypotension, is not a common problem and is usually the result of shock (see Shock) from a heart attack, acute infection, or blood loss following an accident. Occasionally it may occur in people suffering from Addison's disease, a failure of the adrenal glands. This is extremely rare and can easily be corrected by drug treatment.

Because the maintenance of a correct blood pressure is so important, very sophisticated mechanisms have evolved in the body to stabilize it. In the West, the level of general stress, however, has led to

Blood pressure can be tested quickly and easily at the doctor's office.

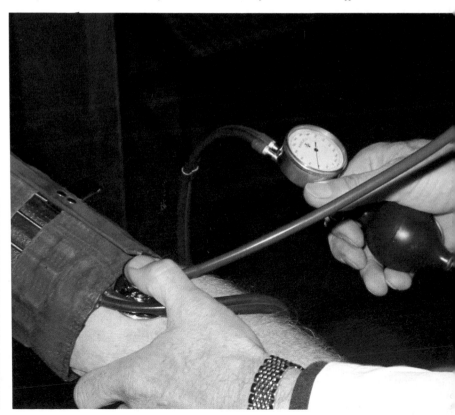

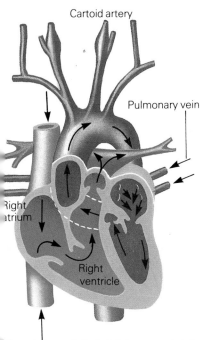

Cartoid artery

Pulmonary vein

Right atrium

Right ventricle

The minimum (diastolic) pressure is taken when the heart has filled with blood from the head, arms, lungs, and body, and is fully distended.

many people developing a level of blood pressure that is much too high for the continuing good health of the arterial system. When this is not the result of disease elsewhere, this is called essential hypertension. The major long-term effect of high blood pressure is on the arteries of the brain, the heart, and the kidneys, with the eventual likelihood of strokes or heart attacks.

What is normal?

The maximum pressure of each heartbeat, or systole, is called the systolic pressure, and the minimum pressure is called the diastolic pressure. It is these two pressures that are measured in order to determine a person's level of blood pressure. Obviously some figure has to be adopted as "normal." For young and middle-aged adults, a pressure of 120 (systolic) over 80 (diastolic)—written as 120/80—is considered normal; 140/90 is cause for concern, while 160/95 is definitely high and requires treatment.

The difficulty of accurately measuring blood pressure is increased by the fact that it rises with age. This is not the case in primitive communities that are untouched by the industrial way of life. Such people enjoy stable blood pressure throughout their lives; in fact, in some cases it even tends to go down with increasing age.

Blood pressure starts to rise when people adopt a more "developed" way of life. But why does the behavior of blood

pressure change in this way? Currently many experts feel that the reason is stress, and there is a growing body of evidence to support this hypothesis. Studies comparing the degree of stress suffered by air traffic controllers and pilots, for example, showed that the stressed controllers had a significantly higher average blood pressure than did the less-stressed pilots.

The influence of diet

There is a significant difference in the type of food that is eaten by developed

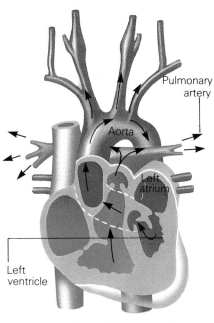

Pulmonary artery

Aorta

Left atrium

Left ventricle

The maximum (systolic) pressure is measured when the heart is pushing the blood out into the body and lungs via the pulmonary artery and the aorta, and they are fully distended.

communities as compared to primitive people. The amount of salt consumed is particularly important, since it has been found that salt tends to increase the volume of blood in circulation, which increases blood pressure. But although the average level of blood pressure in various groups has been found to correspond with their average salt intake, it has been impossible to prove conclusively that higher salt intake necessarily means higher blood pressure. However, it is accepted that both salt intake and stress are among the factors that combine to produce essential hypertension.

Control of hypertension

Whatever the causes may be, the tendency to develop essential hypertension is definitely connected with some kind of overactivity of the normal control mechanisms of the body.

There is an area in the lower part of the brain called the vasomotor center that controls blood circulation and hence blood pressure. The blood vessels that are responsible for controlling the situation are called arterioles and lie between the small arteries and the capillaries in the blood circuit. The vasomotor center receives information about the level of the blood pressure from pressure-sensitive nerves in the aorta (the main artery of the body) and the carotid arteries (to the head) and then sends out instructions to the arterioles through the sympathetic nervous system.

In addition to this fast-acting control, there is also a slower-acting control operating from the kidneys, which are very sensitive to blood flow. When the pressure falls, they release a hormone called renin, which in turn produces a substance called angiotensin. This has two effects: first, it constricts the arterioles and raises the blood pressure; second, it causes the adrenal glands to release a hormone called aldosterone, which makes the kidneys retain salt and causes the blood pressure to rise.

This interaction of the pressure and salt-control systems is an important clue to the cause of essential hypertension, particularly because diuretic pills are widely used in treating high blood pressure. These diuretics (or water pills) cause the kidneys to pass more salt and urine, reducing the volume of the blood and thus bringing down its pressure.

Diagnosis

Raised blood pressure may be the result of a number of conditions apart from essential hypertension. Many kidney diseases cause high blood pressure. Therefore when a person is suspected of having this problem, their kidneys are usually checked. This is easily done, in most cases, with a single blood and urine test. Only occasionally is it necessary for the person to have a kidney X ray. Much information can also be gained from the patient as well.

The blood test measures the urea in the blood—this is likely to be raised if there are kidney defects. The blood level of various salts (sodium, potassium, and bicarbonate) gives clues to other causes of high blood pressure. The urine is screened for the presence of protein, which also occurs in chronic kidney infection or disease. Many doctors will also perform a cardiogram and chest X ray to see if the raised blood pressure has affected the heart in any way.

If the kidneys are found to be working abnormally, it is possible that the raised blood pressure could be the result of renal (kidney) disease. On the other

How the kidneys control blood pressure

Kidneys secrete renin, which produces angiotensin when pressure is low. This constricts arteries and raises blood pressure.

Simultaneously the adrenal glands produce aldosterone, causing salt retention, which also raises pressure and stops renin production.

Adrenal gland

Blood under low pressure

Kidney

Retention of salt in kidney tubules

Raised blood pressure

Bladder

Renin

Angiotensin

Aldosterone

Constriction of arterioles and raised blood pressure

Venner Artists

Aside from cases of malignant hypertension, symptoms of high blood pressure are not always definite. People may complain of headaches, but this does not necessarily mean that they have hypertension. Dizziness and nose bleeds are also common. But the best guide to the state of your blood pressure is to have it checked regularly, every year or two.

Treatment

It has been shown that drug treatment dramatically improves the prospects of survival for both young and middle-aged people suffering from hypertension. But since no drug is without side effects, doctors must consider very carefully at what point their use is justified. This is particularly difficult with elderly patients, who are much more prone to suffer from the side effects of drugs.

Three main types of drugs are used to treat high blood pressure: diuretics (see Diuretics), which cause salt-loss from the kidneys; beta-blockers, which lower blood pressure and get their name from their effect of blocking the action of adrenaline; and vasodilators, which dilate the blood vessels. There are many other drugs that may be used for people, such as asthmatics or the elderly, who cannot tolerate the side effects of beta-blockers.

Outlook

If a person's high blood pressure is treated, the chances of a stroke are greatly reduced, and the risks of having a heart attack are also lowered considerably. This is the reason why it is so important for people to take the drugs they have been prescribed—even when they are feeling perfectly healthy.

hand, the raised blood pressure can itself cause deterioration in the kidneys. This happens because continuing high blood pressure particularly affects the arterioles, causing their walls to thicken. This obstructs the flow of blood and has an adverse effect on kidney function. Sometimes it may be impossible for the doctor to distinguish between cause and effect. A vicious circle may be set up that maintains, and even accelerates, raised blood pressure.

Essential hypertension accounts for 90 percent or more of people with high blood pressure levels. Most of the remaining sufferers have kidney disease, leaving a few with abnormalities of hormone secretion such as an overproduction of cortisone or adrenaline. Another condition that may cause high blood pressure is excessive secretion of aldosterone by the adrenal gland. Fortunately all these forms of hypertension respond to treatment.

Symptoms

Sometimes by the time people feel it is necessary to see their doctor, their blood pressure is already very high indeed. They may already have had blackouts, a minor stroke, and symptoms such as swollen ankles or shortness of breath. This situation is particularly likely in malignant (or accelerated) hypertension and is fatal if left untreated.

The brain disturbances here are due to an increase in the pressures operating inside the skull and pressing on the brain. This can be detected by examining the eye with a strong light; if there is undue pressure, the central nerve at the back of the eye will look inflamed. Examination of the eye will also provide the doctor with other useful information. For example, small arteries at the back of the eye, which are the only ones that can be seen without an operation, will also show definite signs of hypertension.

Self-help with high blood pressure

- Try to reduce the stress in your life. Much of this is due to worry, frustration, and disappointment. It may not be easy, but if you can deal with the problems causing stress, you can lower your blood pressure
- Cut out smoking; the nicotine in cigarettes is rapidly absorbed into the bloodstream and is known to increase blood pressure
- Keep your weight down. If you are overweight, you are making extra work for your circulatory system. Blood pressure can fall within weeks of excess weight being shed
- Take some kind of regular exercise. Jogging or yoga are excellent, although almost any kind of regular exercise will improve the general health and fitness of your body

Blood transfusion

Q Should I carry an identity tag giving my blood group, in case I need a blood transfusion in an emergency?

A No. Identity tags or bracelets are not necessary unless you have a rare blood group or your blood contains antibodies that do not conform to type. Your blood group is always checked before you are given a transfusion. This procedure only takes a couple of minutes.

Q I have been told that the baby I am expecting may need an exchange transfusion. Will there by any problems afterward?

A Not if the baby is otherwise normal. The only difference is that your baby will spend a few days after the transfusion in an incubator in the hospital so that the doctors can make sure that all is progressing satisfactorily.

Q Can blood from a donor be infected?

A It could be, but this was not known in the early days of transfusion in the 17th century. The fact that blood can carry infection was only realized much later. Today great care is taken to prevent contamination by bacteria and viruses. This starts with the donor, who is screened before being allowed to give blood. The blood packs are sterilized during manufacturing and used only once. Strict precautions are taken during storage, and the blood is kept at the right temperature to discourage the growth of bacteria. A final check is given before transfusion.

Q My baby was born by cesarean section, and I was given a blood transfusion during the operation. Am I in danger of getting AIDS through the blood that I was given?

A No. This was a problem in the past, especially for hemophiliacs. Now all donated blood is screened for AIDS antibodies before being used, and high-risk groups are discouraged from donating it in the first place.

Hundreds of thousands of lives are saved every year by blood transfusions, which replace the vital serum and plasma lost in accidents or through disease.

Blood transfusions are not new, but they only became a safe, effective medical treatment in the latter half of the 20th century.

Most people think that transfusions are only used as part of life-saving treatment in accidents and emergencies. But while they are vital in these situations, there are many other reasons for giving a transfusion of blood.

Blood transfusion is a form of tissue transplantation and, as such, it carries certain hazards. Doctors do not advise a transfusion without careful consideration. However, because they are aware of the possible complications, great care is taken in preparing and giving the transfusion to prevent the recipient from suffering side effects. Further limits are imposed by the availability of blood. As this can only be obtained from donors, and as there is often a shortage of donors, care has to be taken to use limited supplies wisely.

Reasons for transfusion

Blood must be replaced when a person suffers an acute blood loss. When this happens, the patient will go into shock due to the loss of circulating blood, and the tissues will be starved of oxygen because of the loss of red cells. Aside from accidents and bleeding during or after childbirth, surgical operations are the usual reason for acute blood loss. Some operations, such as cardiac surgery or a hip replacement, will routinely require a blood transfusion to be given, but a transfusion is only required in most surgery if the case proves more difficult than usual.

A patient with a bleeding duodenal ulcer, prolonged heavy periods, or an infestation of hookworms can lose up to 3.4 fl oz (100 ml) of blood a day. Because this loss is chronic, it sometimes passes unnoticed until the patient becomes very anemic. In this case transfusion may be the only safe way of quickly treating the anemia so that the underlying cause can be cured. A concentration of red cells, rather than normal blood, is used to lessen the danger of overloading the circulation.

Patients with blood conditions like aplastic anemia or thalassemia require repeated transfusions and even white cell and/or platelet transfusions.

Antibody problems

Occasionally patients will make antibodies against their own blood, which leads to its destruction. A blood transfusion

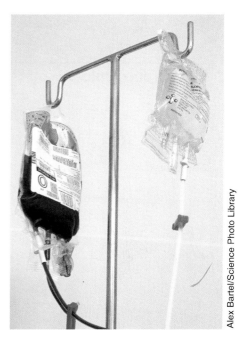

Blood is delivered to the patient by means of an intravenous drip.

may then be required to replace the blood that has been destroyed.

In a condition called hemolytic disease of the newborn, antibodies in the mother's blood attack the baby's blood (as in severe cases of Rhesus disease). When this happens, there is not only a need to replace the red cells that have been destroyed, but there is also a need to remove the offending antibodies from the baby's blood. This process, called exchange transfusion, involves removing a small volume of the baby's blood and replacing it with an equal volume of fresh donor blood. The procedure is repeated until the total volume of the newborn child's blood has been exchanged.

An exchange transfusion is usually performed within hours of the baby's birth, when the blood vessels in the umbilical cord can still be opened. This allows a catheter (a tube) to be introduced into the umbilical artery. The process is painless, and it is usually preferable to putting a needle into one of the baby's delicate veins.

Blood grouping

Blood that has been processed is delivered to a hospital, where it is stored in special blood bank refrigerators. These are

How the analyst works out which group your blood belongs to

	agglutinates with anti-A?	agglutinates with anti-B?
Group A	Yes	No
Group B	No	Yes
Group AB	Yes	Yes
Group O	No	No

Group O blood is the only group that is acceptable to all other groups

Group A blood   Group B blood

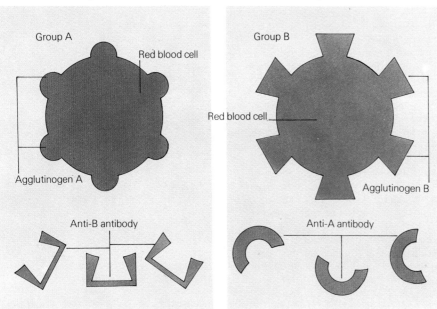

Groups A and B blood contain antibodies that agglutinate (stick together) with red cells from the opposite group if these two incompatible blood types are mixed.

Bernard Fallon

Cross-matching

Once suitable packs of blood have been chosen, they will be cross-matched in the laboratory. This is done by mixing the patient's plasma (which contains antibodies) with red cells from the donor's blood. If the patient's plasma contains antibodies that attack the antigens in the red cells of the donor's blood, the cells will either clump together (agglutinate) or burst (lysis). In this case, the cross-match is said to be incompatible and that unit of blood cannot be given. The process is repeated until sufficient compatible units are found. The compatible units are then carefully labeled and placed in a special section of the blood bank.

Having a transfusion

When the blood is ready for transfusion, the doctor will use a drip to give the patient the blood. The most convenient site is in the lower arm, although other sites can be used.

The doctor will put a tourniquet around the arm, slide a needle into a vein and attach a special set of tubing that incorporates a filter and a flow chamber to insure that the blood does not flow too fast. Initially saline (a salt solution) or some other transfusion fluid will be used to check that the drip is working well, but when it is clear that there are no snags, the doctor will send for the blood. This is carefully checked, and having insured that the unit has definitely been cross-matched for the patient, the pack is attached to the drip tubing and the blood transfusion is under way.

designed to keep the blood within the temperature range of 39–42°F (4–6°C) so that it suffers no deterioration. Before a patient undergoes a blood transfusion, the doctor takes a small sample of his or her blood. This is sent to the laboratory so that suitable blood from a donor can be cross-matched.

First the patient's blood will be grouped. Under ideal conditions he or she will be given a transfusion of blood of the same group, but if the exact match is not available, blood that is of a compatible group will be chosen. The analyst knows that it is important to choose blood where the antibodies already present in the recipient's plasma (the colorless part of blood in which red and white cells float) will not attack and destroy the donor red cells. For example, Group O blood, which has no foreign proteins or antigens (which cause allergic reactions) to stimulate the production of antibodies, can be given to anyone, whereas AB blood will be destroyed by anti-A or anti-B factors and therefore can be given only to an AB recipient.

What would happen if blood Groups A and B were combined

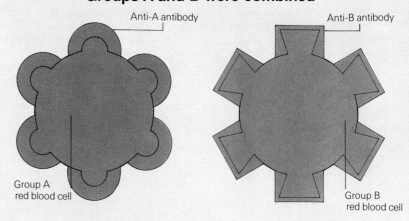

Antibodies from incoming blood combine with the recipient's red blood cells, and antibodies already in the recipient's blood combine with incoming red blood cells, resulting in clotting. This situation almost never happens because blood is carefully cross-matched.

Blue baby

Q My first child was a blue baby. Will any further children I have suffer from the same thing?

A Ask your doctor if this happened because of an inherited heart abnormality. If so, any other children you have may have a slightly greater chance of inheriting the same condition. Otherwise you are no more likely to have another blue baby than is someone whose first child was normal.

Q My aunt had a blue baby that was born a month ahead of time. Are all blue babies premature?

A Although many blue babies are premature, babies who are full term can also suffer from heart conditions that cause blueness. Prematurity may cause a baby to be blue if the ductus arteriosus, which normally connects the pulmonary artery to the aorta, remains open after birth.

Q One doctor at the hospital told me that my child was a blue baby; another that he had a hole in his heart; and yet a third that he had a ventricular septal defect. How can I have any confidence in the treatment if none of them agree?

A You don't have to worry; the doctors do agree. The doctor who told you that your baby was suffering from a ventricular septal defect gave you the correct medical definition. The others are common descriptive names of no medical value that give you a general idea of the condition and one of its outstanding symptoms: the blue color of your baby.

Q My baby is a blue baby, but the doctor won't operate on the hole in his heart. Isn't it dangerous to leave it like this?

A Many holes in the heart close spontaneously during the first year of life. Your doctor probably feels that this will happen in your baby's case. It is always better to wait for a while than to perform unnecessary surgery.

A blue baby is one born with a heart defect. Surgery may be required in some cases; in others the defect may correct itself naturally.

Babies born with congenital heart defects—which are known collectively as holes in the heart—can either have a healthy natural color or purplish-blue lips and skin. The latter condition is called cyanosis, and the characteristic color of the blue baby occurs because there is insufficient oxygen in the blood to change blue blood to red.

Causes

In normal circulation oxygen is extracted from the blood by the body's tissues, and as the blood circulates around the body, it turns blue in color. The blood returns to the heart and enters a collecting chamber called the right atrium, from which it travels to a second chamber called the right ventricle. It is then carried to the lungs, where it receives fresh oxygen and is cleansed of carbon dioxide. This restores the red color to the blood.

The blood then flows to the left atrium and into the left ventricle, from where it is pumped into the body. The action of the blood moving through the lungs from the right side to the left is called pulmonary circulation; the movement of the blood from the left side of the heart, around the body and back to the right side of the heart is called systemic circulation.

A congenital heart defect allows blue blood from the veins to pass through the heart and out to the body again without absorbing oxygen from the lungs. Any abnormality of the heart or blood vessels that allows one-third or more of the systemic flow to consist of unoxygenated blue blood will cause a purplish blue skin color to appear in the baby, and this is present from birth.

The abnormality can consist of a hole between the left and right atria or left and right ventricles, narrow openings to the chambers, or a mix-up between the great vessels that take blood to and from the heart. A child may have one or a combination of these abnormalities, each condition having a different medical name. The two that most commonly produce blueness, however, are called ventricular septal defect and tetralogy of Fallot. Together they account for a third of all congenital heart abnormalities.

Only about one out of every thousand live babies born will have a congenital heart defect. It is not fully known why

The best way to establish the size and location of a blue baby's hole in the heart is by taking an X ray. It can then be decided whether surgery is necessary.

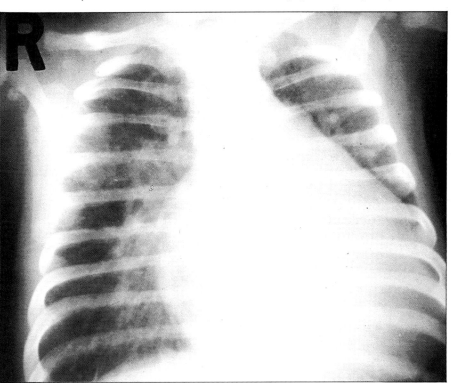

The passage of blood through a heart with a septal defect

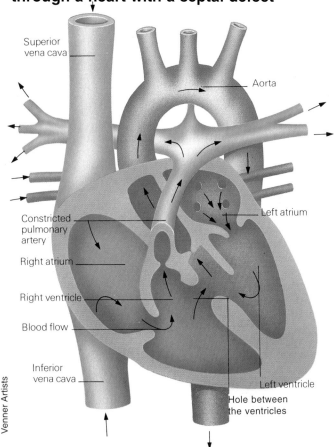

Superior vena cava

Aorta

Constricted pulmonary artery

Left atrium

Right atrium

Right ventricle

Blood flow

Inferior vena cava

Left ventricle

Hole between the ventricles

Venner Artists

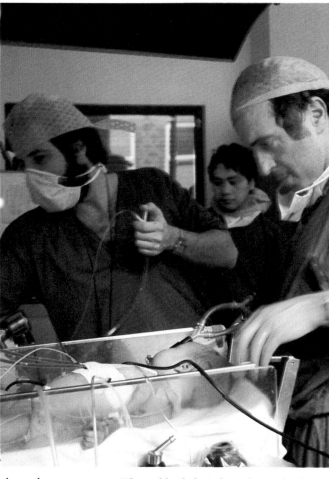

When a blue baby is born, he or she may have problems with breathing and maintaining a stable body temperature. The baby will be placed in an incubator until further investigations can be carried out.

some children are born with defective hearts, but in some cases it is thought there may be a hereditary link. Exposure to rubella (German measles; see Rubella) during the first three months of pregnancy can affect a baby's heart, while certain drugs and other viral infections are other possible causes of abnormality.

Symptoms

Some babies with a heart defect may never look blue, while in others the blueness may develop later if the defect has resulted in an abnormal heart function.

Other symptoms of heart abnormality include experiencing difficulty during swallowing or crying, susceptibility to respiratory infections (such as bronchitis or pneumonia), and a slow recovery afterward. Lack of weight gain and muscular development, and the presence of finger swelling (clubbing) are also symptomatic of a heart defect.

To diagnose an abnormality, the chest is X-rayed to show heart size. An electrocardiograph (a test that measures the activity of the heart muscle) is used to assess the size of the chambers and the thickness of the walls, and other painless, nonsurgical tests are made to assess the amount and direction of blood flow.

A blue baby is likely to have one or more of these tests carried out within the first few days or weeks of life in order to determine whether surgery is necessary for the condition. Other babies with heart abnormalities whose color is normal are often not investigated until they are three or four years old or until doctors think they should be operated on. The decision to operate depends on whether heart failure is anticipated.

Treatment

Each abnormality that causes blueness has a different form of treatment, and operations can be performed at different ages: soon after birth, when the child is a toddler, at preschool age, or even later. The decision whether or not to operate depends both on the condition of the child and the professional opinion of the surgeon.

The most common abnormality that requires surgery is a ventricular septal defect, a hole between the left and right ventricles. The operation to correct it, which carries a mortality rate of less than 5 percent, consists of opening the ventricle and stitching up the hole or putting a plastic patch over it if it is too large to be closed.

Outlook

Once the operation has been performed it is necessary to follow up on the patient for some time to make sure that the heart and lungs are still functioning normally. However, it is generally agreed that if the heart can stand the strain of the defect for the first year of life, it will probably work well for years to come. Many children have gone on to lead a normal life without the need for drugs or further treatment after convalescence.

It is wrong to overprotect children with a heart defect. With very few exceptions, they usually have an instinctive knowledge of how much physical activity they can take. Parents should allow them to decide their own level of activity: their own sensations are a reliable guide. A heart abnormality is not a disease: the muscle is usually strong, and the valves tend to be normal and function well. Therefore the normal running and playing activities that most children enjoy should do no harm.

Blushing

Q I turn red in the face when I eat hot peppers. Is this the same as blushing?

A No. Hot peppers and other spicy foods have this effect on many people, as do alcohol, heat, and sexual arousal. It is one of the body's ways of cooling itself down, and it is called flushing. A flush can last for up to an hour, while a blush—which stems from emotional causes—is usually over in minutes.

Q Whenever I have to speak to a large group, I can't stop blushing. Would it be better to just avoid these situations?

A No. You will lose the habit sooner if you get accustomed to circumstances that you find awkward or embarrassing. It helps to concentrate on what you want to say rather than on how you look when you say it.

Q How can I become less self-conscious when I meet strangers?

A Try to concern yourself with putting the other person at ease, and remember that if people seem standoffish, it may be that they are shy, too, and do not wish to show their vulnerability.

Q Is there anything that I can do to increase my self-confidence?

A Rehearse in your mind every day all your achievements, however small, and firmly chalk up the things that went wrong to experience. It is a natural human tendency to exaggerate the importance of the qualities we lack and belittle those we have—so try to keep things in perspective, and you will find that you gradually become more confident.

Q Why do I blush more in winter than in summer?

A The main reason is that a blush shows up more on a pale winter face than on suntanned skin. Also we tend to sit next to fires or radiators in winter, which causes the skin to flush.

Blushes have an unfortunate way of occurring when we least want them to—when we are embarrassed or angry, for example. But what are the physical causes?

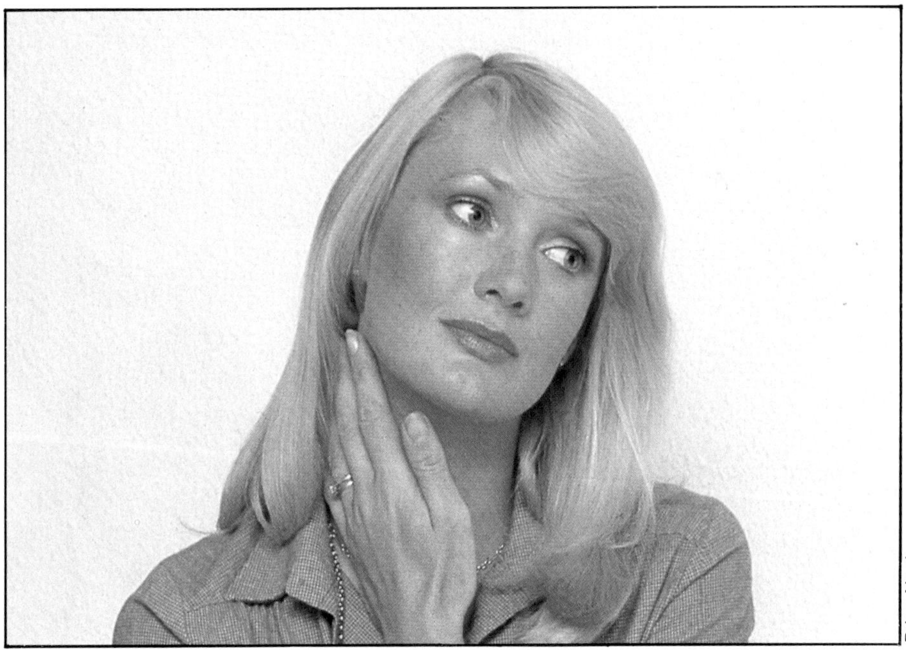

Brian Noah

Everyone knows what it feels like to blush. A sensation of warmth and of blood rushing to the surface spreads from the neck all over the face. It is often accompanied by a quicker heartbeat, tense muscles, a prickling sensation, sweat on the forehead, and a strong urge to hide the face.

Fortunately this event only lasts for a minute or two, and for most people it does not happen often enough to be a nuisance. But a few people blush very easily, and this can be a misery.

Emotional alert

Blushing generally occurs only on exposed areas such as the face and neck. It is usually set off by an unwanted or unexpected feeling or thought that catches a person off guard.

The part of the brain that controls emotion reacts by telling the body to pump out adrenaline and prepare for action. This causes some of the blood vessels near the skin's surface to relax. They then dilate as extra blood flows into them. This shows through the skin as a rosy glow.

Blushing tendencies

Some people are more prone to blushing than others. Women blush more easily than men, and the hot flashes of menopause (when women cease to menstruate) have no counterpart in the middle-aged male.

A blush is more obvious in a fair-skinned person, especially a redhead, than in people with more pigment (coloring) in their skin. Adolescents are very susceptible, because they tend to be very self-conscious at this stage in their physical and social development.

Shy people blush more than those who are self-confident and extroverted, and some elderly people blush frequently if they are suffering from loss of confidence as a result of the aging process and social pressures put on them.

Inner turmoil

The emotional triggers to blushing include: a feeling that a person may look or sound silly; a fear of disapproval; anxiety; anger; and shame or guilt. It is even possible to blush when experiencing secret thoughts and desires.

Mind over matter

It is impossible to control the physical mechanism that causes blushing. But it is possible to reduce the number of situations that make one feel like blushing.

Practice in handling social situations and exercises to increase confidence are the best ways to do this. For the few who blush excessively, medication may prove useful. Most people grow out of this habit by their mid-20s and no special treatment is necessary. But the ability to blush occasionally can show a refreshing sensitivity.

Body language

Q No one ever approaches me at a party. I am really fed up with being a wallflower. How can I meet and talk to new people, especially boys?

A You may be giving out the wrong signals. First talk to and stand near the people you do know. If you sit in a corner on your own, it will look like you are not interested. Check your posture—if you are nervous and tense, your head may slump forward and your arms may be folded defensively across your chest. It is better to hold your head up and let your arms rest naturally at your sides. If you see someone you like, make brief eye contact, smile, then look away. The other person will get the message that you find him or her interesting and can decide whether to respond.

Q My husband is always ready to resent me whenever I ask him to do something. It doesn't seem to matter what I say—he's in a huff even before the words are out of my mouth. What can I do to make him listen?

A You cannot force anyone to listen. However, you can make it easier for your husband. If you expect him to sulk, chances are you will stand defiantly with arms crossed while he sits down. Automatically this will make him feel threatened. Try sitting calmly in a chair—nearby, but not directly across from him, as a face-to-face position often nurtures a confrontation. Let your hands relax in your lap with the palms upward—this will indicate that you are open to his response. Keep your voice even and pleasant. You will probably find that you get a better reception with this behavior.

Q Why do female models in fashion magazine ads always seem to have their mouths hanging open?

A They have probably been told to do so by the photographer. Lips that are wet and slightly parted mimic the female genitals, giving an unconscious signal of sexual availability. This can help to sell the product being represented.

Body language is a system of nonverbal communication that is used by people in all cultures. By learning the meaning behind the most commonly used gestures, a better understanding of friends, family, and others with whom we interact can be achieved.

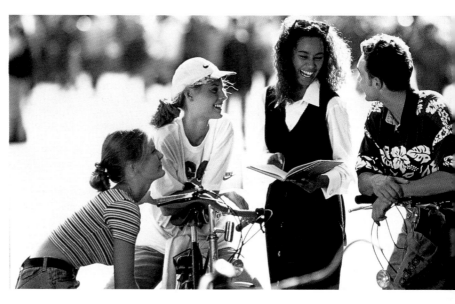

The gestures and movements that people make with their bodies are called body language. During the course of a day, more than 90 percent of face-to-face communication is nonverbal. Most of the knowledge we gain about other people is unconscious—and we may be much better at deciphering body signals than we realize, as an automatic process of assessment occurs.

During the first few moments of meeting someone new, their eye movements, facial expressions, changes in posture, standing or sitting positions, and even clothing, all convey important information about their thoughts, feelings, background, and self-image—and our own body language gives the other person equally important information about us. We decide, almost instantly, whether we like or dislike someone, and we make judgments about their intelligence, personality, suitability as a friend or a lover, and so on. First impressions are very important—and generally, they are long lasting.

Eye contact

One of the most powerful forms of body language is eye contact. This type of contact is usually made to communicate interest, invite interaction with someone, influence (or threaten) others, or provide feedback during the normal course of a conversation.

Groups of friends often copy or mirror each other's postures and gestures as an unconscious display of trust, companionship, and belonging.

There are unspoken rules and regulations regarding a mutual gaze, which vary in different situations. For example, it is usually considered highly rude to stare at strangers or even to look at them in some cases. On the other hand, a parent and child may engage in more or less constant eye contact combined with touching or body contact, and lovers often engage in long, lingering looks that convey their mutual feeling of love and affection.

An example of unacceptable eye contact is the big city rush-hour scenario where people are squashed together in a crowded train. In this situation it is considered an affront to make eye contact that lasts more than a fleeting moment. Any longer than that and a definite hostility may be felt by the person being stared at.

There are several reasons why a person may find it uncomfortable to be watched in a public place: they may feel threatened in some way; they may think the watcher is interested in them sexually; or they may simply be self-conscious about how they look or how their actions make them appear to other people.

Universal gestures

Although body language may vary from country to country, some gestures have been found to be universally shared by all people. The smile is one such gesture. It is a sign of friendship and happiness that crosses all boundaries. Studies of babies who were born deaf and blind have shown that they still smile, proving that it is an inborn trait and not a behavior that needs to be learned. Recent research has found that if a person is feeling depressed or anxious, forcing a smile can actually help to lift the spirits and put him or her in a better mood. Part of the reason for this may be that a smile is usually returned with a smile—a pleasant expression is more attractive to others than a scowling or challenging one and therefore more likely to be answered positively.

The head nod universally signifies acceptance. So if a person were to travel to another country, even if he or she did not know the language, a simple head nod could be used to communicate agreement. Similarly shaking the head from side to side usually signifies disagreement. The shoulder shrug is another such gesture, signaling that a person does not know or understand what is happening.

Hands and arms

The hands and arms can be very expressive. During a conversation, if a person uses hand gestures and their palms are facing upward toward the other person, this gives the impression of an open, honest attitude. Rubbing the palms together can indicate excitement or pleasant expectation of a future event—it is like saying "I can't wait!"

Hands placed together, where the fingers form a steeple, give the impression of a confident attitude, although this can sometimes make the other person feel subordinate or inferior. It is a gesture often used by managers when speaking to their employees or teachers when speaking to their students.

When folded in front of the body, the arms form a barrier to the outside world. This arm-barrier gesture is often used when a person feels threatened or ill at ease in a situation. Younger people tend to fold their arms tighter and closer to their bodies than older people, who have learned to relax more and who may fold their arms in a looser, less obvious way. If the hands are clenched into fists in an arm-barrier position, it indicates a hostile attitude; and if the thumbs stick out and upward, a superior attitude is displayed.

Pointers

The body has a distinct tendency to point in the direction where the mind wants to go. For example, a man and a woman who have just met and are sitting together at a party may be engaged in what sounds like a pleasant conversation. But if the woman's body is turned away from the man, although her head may be tilted slightly toward him as a sign of minimal courtesy, she is not really interested in what he is saying and would like to move away from him as soon as possible.

Legs that are uncrossed and pointed toward the direction of the speaker indicate an open, friendly attitude, whereas crossed legs, in either a sitting or standing position, show varying degrees of defense, displeasure, or closing up. A person standing or sitting with folded arms and crossed legs is in the ultimate defensive position—he or she is literally putting up as many physical barriers as possible.

Proximity and position

The amount of space a person needs around them in order to feel comfortable when interacting with others can vary. Edward Hall, who called this study of personal space proxemics, described four main zones of varying intimacy.

The intimate zone, which would only be available to closest friends and family, is from zero to one-and-a-half feet (0 to 0.5 m). The personal zone extends from one-and-a-half to four feet (0.5 to 1.2 m) and allows others to be kept at arm's length.

Everyday social and business contact is conducted in the social-consultive zone, from four to ten feet (1.2 to 3 m), and finally the public zone, which covers all other human contact, extends from ten feet (3 m) outward.

People who have grown up in the country, where there are plenty of wide, open spaces, tend to need a lot more personal space, or territory, than those brought up in the more cramped, crowded conditions of a big city. Likewise those brought up in an urban environment may feel uncomfortable when confronted with too much space and too few people.

Positioning in face-to-face communication is important. At a table, placing two people directly across from each other is likely to provoke competitive or combative feelings. Diagonal seating puts both parties more at ease, especially in an interviewing situation.

Although eye contact is more difficult, side-by-side seating is the most intimate, because some physical contact is unavoidable. This tends to enhance cooperation in business situations and

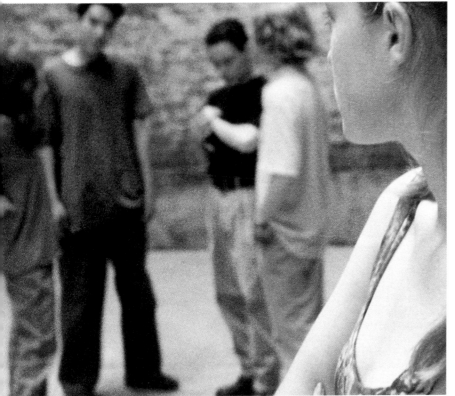

The direction in which the feet are pointing indicates real interest. This teenage boy (left) is talking to his male friends, but his feet are pointing toward the girl in the foreground.

Q My two-year-old son cocks his head so far sideways while he is having a conversation that he looks as though he will fall over. Is this normal?

A Yes, it is. Young children often use this gesture when they are listening intently. Look around at the other adults and children with whom he has regular contact—he may be exaggerating their poses. At any rate, children usually modify the gesture as they get older, so it becomes less obvious.

Q I have a job interview coming up, and I'd really like to get the job. Are there body language techniques I can use to help my chances?

A Yes, there are things you can do to make a good impression, and first impressions are always important. Before you arrive at the interview, take a few deep breaths to relax. Keep your posture straight and your head erect but not stiff as you walk into the room. As you sit in your chair, lean forward slightly—this will show you are interested. If you sit back in the chair and get too comfortable, the interviewer may think that you are arrogant or feel you are too good for the job. Let your arms sit naturally in your lap, keeping your hands open when gesturing—the palms-upward position is always interpreted as a friendly sign. Smile often but not constantly. And, of course, don't forget to answer the interviewer's questions!

Q I have just started dating a woman who is a few inches taller than me; she is constantly crouching, with her head hanging down, when we go out together. Why does she bother?

A She may be self-conscious about appearing taller than you. Traditionally men were supposed to be the bigger-and-stronger sex. Your new friend is trying to make you feel that you are taller so that you will feel protective and not threatened by her. Try to reassure her that you find her—and her height—attractive.

Body contact—touching

The behavior of touching is sometimes called haptics. The term *touching* assumes that the act is deliberate and consciously performed, usually using the hands. Below is a list, prepared by Michael Argyle (who wrote a book called *Bodily Communication*), of the most common ways that people touch each other in Western cultures. The degree of touching varies according to the level of intimacy experienced between two people.

Shaking: Hands
Patting: Head, back
Stroking: Hair, face
Kissing: Mouth, cheek, hand
Licking: Face
Holding: Hand, arm
Embracing: Shoulder, body
Slapping: Face, hand, bottom

Punching: Face, chest
Pinching: Cheek
Linking: Arms
Laying-on: Hands
Kicking: Bottom
Grooming: Hair, face
Tickling: Anywhere

In addition the anthropologist Desmond Morris identified body contact in a sexual manner with these 12 steps to sexual intimacy. Western couples in love almost always follow this order of touching, from first glance to full intimacy.

1	Eye to body		7	Mouth to mouth
2	Eye to eye		8	Hand to head
3	Voice to voice		9	Hand to body
4	Hand to hand		10	Mouth to breast
5	Arm to shoulder		11	Hand to genitals
6	Arm to waist		12	Genitals to genitals

also may enhance a feeling of sexual attraction between two people at a social gathering.

Mirroring

When one person is listening intently to another, there is a tendency for the listener to copy the movements of the speaker; this is a way of saying "I understand and agree with you" or "we really do think alike." By using this system of mirroring (or carbon copying, as it is sometimes called) another person's gestures, a person is seeking to gain their acceptance in some way.

For example, an employer who is trying to be on the same level as his or her employee may mimic the way the employee is sitting across the desk. In the course of a conversation, if the employee folds his or her hands on the table, the employer will do the same. If he or she scratches his face, the action will be copied. In this way subservience (with possible ulterior motives behind it) is shown by the employer.

By studying mirroring gestures, it is easy to tell which person in a couple or group is the decision maker. For example, although the man in a married couple may be doing all the talking in a social situation, if the woman is making gestures and the man is watching and then mirroring these, she is likely to be the unspoken leader of the two. Similarly the leader of a group often makes silent motions to other, more vocal group members known to be under his or her influence—and these gestures are immediately responded to.

Synchronized gestures

In many mirroring situations a kind of synchronicity is established where similar movements are made roughly at the same time.

This gestural synchrony, as it is called, is used to an even greater degree in friendships, where it signals a sense of belonging and kinship, and in romantic relationships, where a growing sense of understanding and affection is developing between the parties.

A display of copied or mirrored gestures, when it is combined with synchronized timing, is a definite sign of interest between two people who have just met and are attracted to each other in some way. It is a positive way of creating a feeling of trust.

Speech signals

Just as gestures can change to mirror other people's, patterns of speech and tone of voice may also be modified with each new interaction. A person may match the volume, voice quality (i.e. soft or harsh), speed of speech, and even the accent of another person in a conversation. This kind of mirroring has the effect of putting the other person at ease and creating a feeling of mutual

The face often gives universal clues as to what a person is feeling. This man (right) is obviously experiencing either great pain or disappointment.

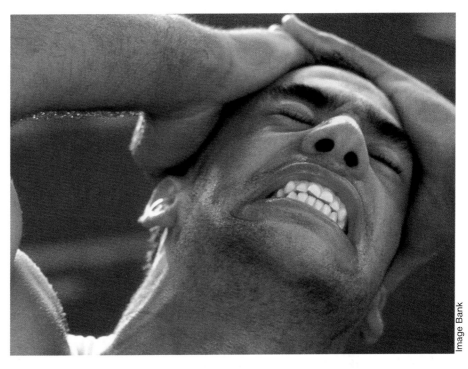

Image Bank

trust, because again it is a way of saying "we are alike."

A consistently loud voice may give the impression that a person wishes to dominate, whereas a soft voice may indicate a submissive personality. The stress placed on certain words also matters—a slight rise in volume on affirmative words, such as *yes* and *great*, rather than on negative words, such as *no* and *never*, will create a much more positive impression. Speed of speech is also important; fast talkers are sometimes perceived as being untrustworthy.

Physical appearance

The type of clothing a person may choose to wear, including details such as color, style, and era of clothing, i.e., brand-new or secondhand, can also reveal a lot about the personality, age, background, and status of an individual, and how they want to be perceived.

Many people tend to adhere to current fashions, and assumptions are made if there is any discrepancy from the norm. A general rule is that the more individual the clothing, the less the wearer is interested in looking like everybody else for whatever reason—be it neglect, rebellion, disinterest, or unusual preferences.

Clothing and hairstyles are closely tied to the social group that a person wishes to be associated with. Conservative members of society, such as Republican politicians, may be careful to appear in public always well-dressed in classic suits and dresses, with traditionally styled hair and perfect makeup.

On the other hand, an artistic person, such as a painter or a rock star, may wear unusual or quirky clothing of clashing colors and have a wild, unkempt hairstyle. People who wish to be seen as artistic may copy them.

It is possible to change dramatically the way that others perceive you by wearing different clothes. Over a long period of time any new image you project will tend to alter your own self-image, because people will react to you in a different way.

Outlook

The study of body language in humans and other animals has existed from ancient times and is in a continual state of change. New sciences are being developed for all of its different aspects.

By learning about the impression you make on others, it is possible to modify your own body language, to increase your understanding of human nature, and to use this knowledge in both personal and professional situations to better interpersonal relations.

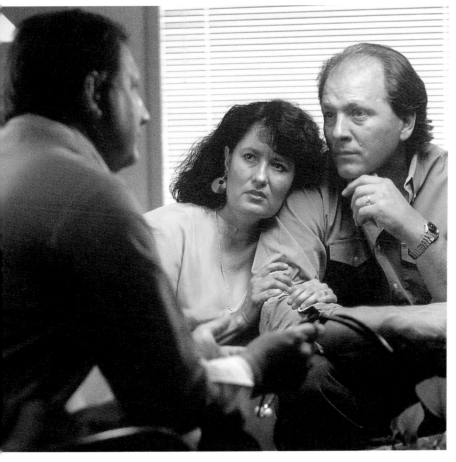

Competitive or confrontational situations often occur when people are seated opposite each other, as with these two men. The woman shows her support by gripping the man protectively.

Body odor

Q I never know whether to buy a deodorant or an antiperspirant. Which is best?

A A deodorant contains a pleasant-smelling chemical that masks the odor of sweat, while antiperspirants actually reduce the evaporation of the sweat so that the odor is sealed in. Try a deodorant first, and if this does not control the odor, then try an antiperspirant. Both are perfectly safe to use.

Q I've noticed that children don't seem to suffer from body odor. Why is this?

A Children's sweat is not so different from adult sweat, but they do have smaller bodies that sweat less. Also they have no underarm hair to trap stale sweat. Children still smell when they sweat heavily, however, as any gym teacher will know. The odor is slightly metallic but not unpleasant.

Q Is perspiration just another word for sweat?

A Yes, but perspiration generally describes moderate sweating, which is a steady production of sweat that does not form into heavy droplets on the skin.

Q Why do some people seem to sweat more than others?

A The mechanism of sweating is controlled by the nerves and is affected by both a person's excitability and the state of the skin's blood vessels. Every person is different. For example, heavier people have to sweat more to cool themselves off, and anxious people sweat more because their nerves are more active.

Q I've heard that women find men's body odor attractive. How can this be?

A When the smell is mild, it can be sexually attractive. Sweat contains substances that, in animals anyway, are used for sexual signals. Humans may react unconsciously in the same way, but odor can soon become offensive, so personal hygiene is a safe bet.

Most of us worry about body odor. In fact, everyone has an individual smell, but it is what a person does about this odor that determines whether or not it becomes offensive.

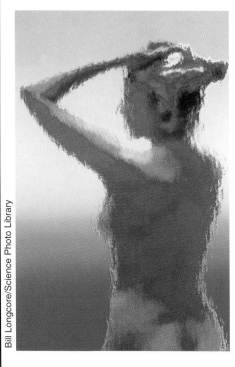

Bill Longcore/Science Photo Library

The best way to prevent odor is regular, thorough bathing or showering.

Body odor is caused by sweat. And sweat, or perspiration, is important in regulating the body's temperature, because its evaporation from the skin has a cooling effect.

Perspiration

The sweat glands—of which humans have about two million—can produce up to 6 pints (2.8 liters) of perspiration in one day. Sweat consists mostly of water and salt, with a small amount of waste products. It has very little odor in itself, and only begins to smell unpleasant when it becomes old and stale and the skin's bacteria begin to act upon it.

Sweat from some parts of the body is much more likely to cause an odor than from others. This sweat, called apocrine sweat, is produced by the sweat glands in the armpits and around the genitals and anus, and it is thicker than perspiration from the rest of the body.

Individual differences

Sweating varies from person to person and from time to time. Some people sweat so little that it is virtually unnoticeable, while others have to contend with very active sweat glands.

Sweating increases with exercise and also with nervous tension. On a cool day a person may hardly sweat at all, while on a hot day the sweat glands work overtime. If the air is very humid, it prevents the sweat from evaporating, which is why one may feel so sticky and uncomfortable.

Abnormal perspiration

Very pungent body odor can occasionally be due to a serious medical condition or skin infection. Certain diseases can cause excessive sweating, while in some medical conditions sweating is reduced to a minimum. A few people suffer from hyperhidrosis—increased sweating—which requires medical treatment.

How often to wash

The best way to keep body odor under control is to follow a careful personal hygiene routine that includes regular washing of clothing as well as the body. A bath or shower once a day is the ideal solution. Washing more frequently can disturb healthy skin bacteria and make odor problems even worse.

Shaving the armpits does not reduce sweat—but it does reduce the amount of trapped sweat that might otherwise become stale and produce offensive odor. Deodorants and antiperspirants can never remove body odor, but they can help to control it by reducing apocrine sweat.

How to prevent body odor

- Bathe or shower daily, especially after exercise, to prevent a buildup of sweat
- Shave under your arms if you are female so that sweat cannot become trapped in the hair
- Dry thoroughly, using a clean towel that is not too soft—a slightly rough surface is more effective
- Keep the use of scented talcum powder or perfume to a minimum. These can combine with sweat or bacteria to produce a stale odor
- Apply deodorant or antiperspirant regularly if you sweat heavily
- Wash sweaters, shirts, underwear, pants, and other clothing regularly
- Wear comfortable, loose clothing in hot weather
- Wear cotton underwear, which lets the skin breathe more than nylon

Body structure

Q Aside from the obvious sexual differences, do men and women differ in their actual body structures? And, if so, how great are the differences?

A On average, men are 6 in (15 cm) taller than women and show quite a number of internal differences in body structure. Most men have larger hearts and lungs than women and are made of 42 percent muscle, compared with 36 percent in women. A man's body contains about 4 percent more water than a woman's. This is because a woman's body has more fat beneath the skin, and fat is a water-free substance.

Q Is it true that some people have their appendix on the wrong side?

A Yes, some people are born with their appendix on the left rather than the right side of the body, and there are many other odd variations in body structure. For example, babies may be born with a bottom rib missing, with extra fingers and toes, or with a webbing of skin between their fingers or toes. Most of these conditions can be surgically corrected.

Q My husband and I are both much taller than average. Does this mean that our son will be tall too?

A Unlike other details of the body's structure, such as eye color, a person's height is governed not only by inheritance factors, or genes, but also by the effects of environment. Your son will probably be taller than average, but his final height will also depend on his diet and the proper functioning of many of his internal organs. However many genes for tallness he inherits, your son will not grow properly if his diet is deficient in proteins or the mineral calcium, which is needed for building bones. Even with a perfect diet, his growth would be retarded if he had something wrong with his supply of the growth hormone, somatrophin. This is a substance that is necessary if his body is to be able to use the food he eats for the enlargement of his bones and other internal body structures.

The human body is fascinating to most people, but for a better understanding of the discoveries made about it, a working knowledge of its structure is required.

Structure simply means the way something is put together. In the case of the human body it is possible to talk about an enormously complicated structure by reducing its many parts to a set of very simple labels—this is something like medical shorthand.

Doctors are always having to do this in order to make themselves clear to each other. They may say something about a skeletal defect or problems with the digestive system, but unless the patient understands what a doctor means when he or she speaks, being treated for an illness can be a mystifying experience.

Some of the terms in this basic shorthand are concerned with differences such as race. But most go to make up a picture of what every human body is like—under the skin.

Race

For classification humanity can be divided into three huge groups, or races, namely the Mongoloids, Negroids, and Caucasians. All have certain structural characteristics, and each, in turn, can be divided into many subgroups.

Mongoloids are typified by yellow skin, straight black hair, and eyes with folded lids that give them an almond-shaped appearance. The Mongoloid body has little hair, and the average male height ranges from 5 ft, 2 in (1.57 m) to 5 ft, 8 in (1.73 m). The Chinese and the Inuit are typical Mongoloid types.

Negroids have brown to black skin and woolly hair. Like Mongoloids, their bodies have very little hair, and they have broad noses, although the Mongoloid nose is narrower at the base. Negroids vary in

Body cavities and urinary system

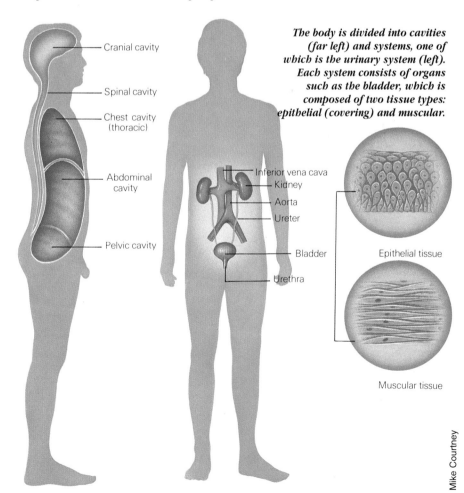

Cranial cavity
Spinal cavity
Chest cavity (thoracic)
Abdominal cavity
Pelvic cavity

Inferior vena cava
Kidney
Aorta
Ureter
Bladder
Urethra

Epithelial tissue

Muscular tissue

The body is divided into cavities (far left) and systems, one of which is the urinary system (left). Each system consists of organs such as the bladder, which is composed of two tissue types: epithelial (covering) and muscular.

BODY STRUCTURE

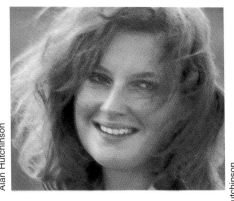

Alan Hutchinson

This Caucasian female has the paleness of the Nordic group of the race.

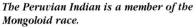

The Peruvian Indian is a member of the Mongoloid race.

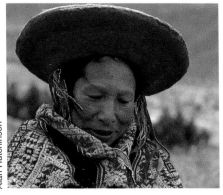

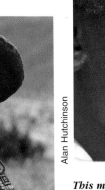

Alan Hutchinson

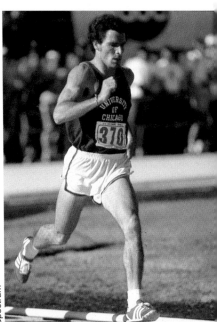

Alan Hutchinson

This man from Nigeria is a Yoruba, one of the many groups of the Negroid race.

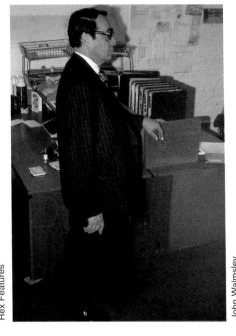

Rex Features

An endomorph tends to have excess body weight and a rounded build.

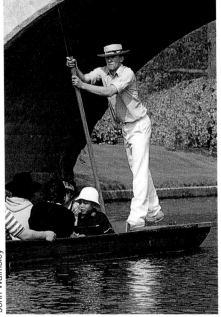

John Walmsley

The ectomorph is lean and angular, but not excessively muscular.

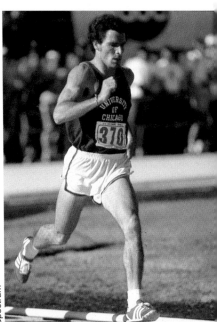

Spectrum

This athlete is a prime example of the muscular mesomorph.

height—from the Bushmen, averaging 4 ft, 8 in (1.42 m) to the Nilotes, whose adult males average 5 ft, 10 in (1.78 m). Most African Americans are classified as Negroids.

Caucasians, the so-called white races of the world, are in fact very mixed, with skin color ranging from brown, as in Indian peoples, to the pale coloring of the Nordic (meaning generally found in the north) subdivisions of the race. Their hair may be any shade of brown, black, red, or blond. The body of a Caucasian male is much more hairy than that of the other two races, and the face and nose are narrower.

One of the least variable Caucasian features is average height, which ranges (for the adult male) from 5 ft, 3 in (1.6 m) in Mediterranean peoples, to 5 ft, 8 in (1.73 m) in Nordic types.

As well as these three major groupings and their subdivisions, there are many mixed, or composite, races.

Shape

All people on Earth can be divided into three groups according to their body shape. The names given these three groups are endomorphs, ectomorphs, and mesomorphs.

A typical endomorph is heavily built and well rounded with a higher than average proportion of body fat and a tendency toward obesity.

The ectomorph is lean and angular with less fat and muscle than average and is capable of a high degree of physical endurance.

The mesomorph is muscular and agile, the typical athlete body shape, and is the strongest of the three.

Of course not everybody conform exactly to this standard pattern—mos people are a mixture of all three types— but each person has an overall leaning to one of the three basic body shapes.

In addition these body types each tend to have a certain behavior pattern Extreme endomorphs tend to be ver relaxed with slow heartbeats and breath ing rates. They are tolerant and good com pany but are inclined to overindulge i food and drink.

The extreme ectomorph is the exac opposite. Hypersensitive and very awar of everything that is happening, he or sh tends to react quickly to new situation But he or she is likely to be obsessive an easily thrown off balance by personal se backs. Between the two is the meso morph, who is typically dominating aggressive, and successful.

Body systems

The body, whatever its race or shape, is divided into four sections—the neck and head; the chest or thoracic cavity, which contains the heart and lungs; the abdomen, housing the alimentary canal, kidneys, liver, and various other organs; and finally the limbs.

To understand how these different parts link up and work together, the body can be studied in systems—groups of organs that work together. One of the most familiar is the digestive system. Others include the nervous and reproductive systems.

Tissues and cells

Each organ is made up of tissues that are made up of cells. The cells are complex collections of chemicals, including such components as the chromosomes that carry the genes, the body's units of inheritance.

Many of the body organs have names that are familiar to us, such as adenoids, appendix, or tongue, but the tissues are less well-known. There are four main types and each organ contains at least one of them.

Epithelial tissues are those that cover or line body organs, and many secrete substances such as hormones (see Hormones). Connective tissues, which include bones and tendons, connect, support, and fill out body structures, including the blood. Muscle tissue enables

What we are made of

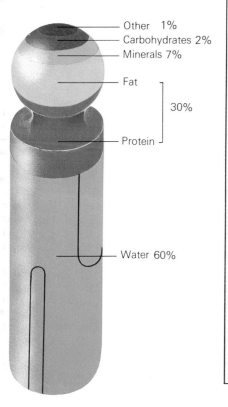

- Other 1%
- Carbohydrates 2%
- Minerals 7%
- Fat
- 30%
- Protein
- Water 60%

movement of the whole body and internal parts. Nervous tissue helps all the body parts to work in harmony by providing communication and control.

Body fluids

About 60 percent of the body is made up of water—but it is not like tap water. Body water contains a huge variety of dissolved salts that make it much more like seawater—where the first living things are known to have evolved. The watery parts of the body are known generally as the body fluids.

A 154 lb (70 kg) man contains on average about 18.5 pints (8.7 liters) of body fluids. Of these, 12.5 pints (5.9 liters) are inside the cells and are called intracellular fluids. The other 6 pints (2.8 liters) outside the cells are called extracellular fluids. Of these, 1.3 pints (0.6 liters) are in the blood plasma—the rest of the blood is made up of cells. The remaining 4.7 pints (2.2 liters) are divided between the interstitial fluid, which bathes the cells and body cavities; the lymph fluid; the fluid around the spine and in the joints; and the fluid in places such as the eyes. All of this fluid is in a constant state of movement in and out of the cells.

The body's fluid is even more important to survival than food. It is essential for carrying oxygen, food substances, and hormones around the body and getting rid of wastes. The body maintains a constant check on its fluid level, and if this level becomes too low, thereby endangering proper body functioning, the water-monitoring center in the brain immediately generates a sensation of thirst, so the person feels the need to drink and rebalance body fluid levels.

A guide to body systems

System	Major organs	Major tissues in typical organ
Digestive	Mouth, teeth, tongue, salivary glands, esophagus (tube from back of throat to stomach), stomach, small and large intestines, anus, liver, gallbladder, pancreas	Stomach—epithelial, muscular
Urinary	Kidneys, ureters (tubes joining the kidneys and bladder), bladder, urethra	Bladder—epithelial, muscular
Muscular	All body muscles, some under conscious control (skeletal or striped muscles), others working unconsciously (smooth muscles)	Biceps muscle—muscular, connective
Skeletal	All the body's bones and the joints that connect them	Connective
Respiratory	Lungs, bronchi (tubes to lungs), trachea (windpipe), mouth, larynx (voice box), nose, diaphragm	Lungs—epithelial, connective
Circulatory	Heart, arteries, veins, capillaries, blood	Heart—muscular
Nervous	Brain, sense organs (eyes, ears, taste buds, smell and touch receptors), nerves, spinal cord	Nervous
Endocrine	Hormone-producing glands: pituitary, thyroid, parathyroid, adrenals, pancreas, thymus, parts of testes and ovaries, and small areas of tissue in the intestine	Pancreas—epithelial, connective
Reproductive (male)	Testes, penis, prostate gland, seminal vesicles, urethra	Penis—muscular, vascular
Reproductive (female)	Ovaries, fallopian tubes, uterus (womb), cervix (neck of womb), vagina	Uterus—muscular, epithelial
Lymphatic	Structures involved in the body's defense against disease, including lymph nodes, lymph vessels, spleen, tonsils, adenoids, thymus (gland in chest)	Spleen—connective, epithelial

Boils

Q I have heard that getting boils repeatedly can be a sign of diabetes. My father has had boils all his life, so could he be diabetic?

A Probably not. It is when boils appear in a person who has not previously had them and who is also generally sick that a doctor will become alarmed and test for diabetes. Your father should definitely have a urine test to make sure, but the fact that he has had boils for many years indicates there is some other cause. Suggest he go to the doctor anyway.

Q I have a small boil on my neck and am very worried that it will leave a scar. Do you think this is likely?

A Small boils on the neck and buttocks will leave tiny scars, but these are not usually noticeable. Some large boils that occur on the face, however, do leave scars, because scar tissue is formed as part of the healing process. These shrink but never disappear entirely.

Q I've heard conflicting advice on whether you should squeeze a boil. Is it ever safe?

A A small boil with a good head of pus can usually be squeezed without danger, but it is wise to be patient and leave it to heal by itself. Never squeeze boils that are very large, multiple boils, or boils with considerable inflammation in the surrounding tissue. This could easily spread infection elsewhere. Never squeeze a boil that is situated between the eye and nose, as spread of infection from this area is potentially dangerous.

Q Can an ordinary pimple turn into a boil?

A Tiny pimples are usually minute abscesses just under the surface of the skin. They occur most commonly as acne. While a boil is also an abscess, it occurs in a hair follicle, which is deep down in the underneath layer of skin. So ordinary pimples will not become boils even if scratched or picked.

Boils are unsightly and sometimes painful, but they will almost always clear up by themselves. However, treatment may be necessary to eliminate any risk of their spreading.

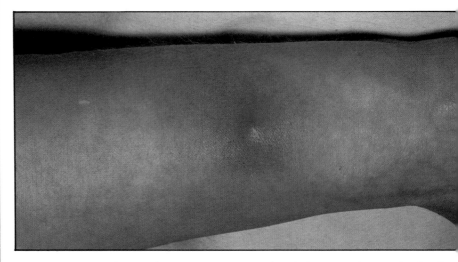

On a young person a boil needs no attention apart from dressing once it bursts.

A carbuncle has more than one head and needs medical treatment.

Hair follicles—a type of pore or tiny pit from which hair grows—lie deep in the lower layer of human skin. If one of these follicles becomes infected by invading bacteria (germs), an abscess, or swelling filled with pus, forms. This type of abscess is commonly called a boil; the medical name is a furuncle.

A carbuncle is two or more boils occurring next to each other, and a boil that forms in one of the hair follicles along the eyelid is called a sty (see Sty).

Location

Boils can occur anywhere on the body, but they appear most often on the face, eyelids, back of the neck, upper back, and buttocks. They especially favor places where clothing rubs, such as the area on the collar line.

Causes

The bacteria known as staphylococci are the most common cause of boils. These bacteria can be transmitted from person to person, and some live harmlessly on the skin all the time. They also thrive in infected areas like cuts or pimples. They usually only cause trouble when excessive friction or rubbing has buried them in a hair follicle.

Infection happens most easily when a person is overworked or anemic or badly undernourished for some reason, as can happen with alcoholism. Some people who eat a very fatty diet may also be prone to boils, for they are probably increasing the greasiness of their skin,

and the infection thrives in greasy blocked-up pores.

Diabetics (see Diabetes) can have a series of boils when their blood-sugar concentration remains high. This is because the bacteria breed fast when there is sugar present in the tissues. And when the skin is broken, as in scabies or eczema, boils develop much more easily.

Symptoms

A boil starts gradually with a tender area under the skin. It becomes hot and red and may be surrounded by swelling.

Pus (see Pus) develops in the center where the fight against the infection is fiercest. It is made up of casualties—dead bacteria, dead white blood cells, and destroyed body tissue. On places like the ear or nose, where the skin is tight and the surrounding tissue cannot stretch, the condition is very painful.

Healing

As soon as the pus from a boil has been released and the central core of dead tissue is gone, the boil heals. This may take about a week. Occasionally the body's defenses will get the best of a boil, and the inflammation will go away without the boil bursting.

Scarring

A small boil will heal without leaving a noticeable scar, but large boils and carbuncles do form scar tissue (see Scars) that may shrink over the months but never disappears altogether.

Common sites of boils

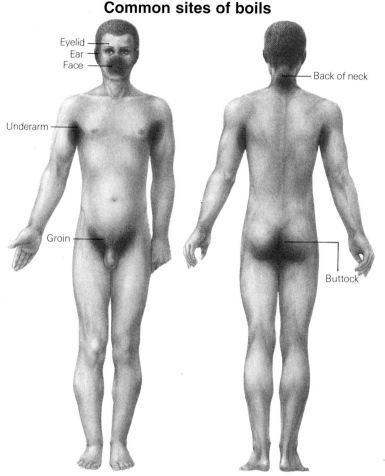

Eyelid
Ear
Face
Underarm
Groin
Back of neck
Buttock

The best way to reduce the likelihood of a large boil or carbuncle scar is to treat the boil as soon as possible. The sooner a person sees the doctor, the quicker he or she will be able to get the boil under control. Many people believe that it is possible to lessen the effects of scarring by rubbing vitamin E cream into the wound, but there is little or no evidence to support this.

The main danger from a boil is that the infection may enter the bloodstream and spread around the body. Boils occurring around the eyes and nose are particularly dangerous, because their poison could spread to the brain.

Special care
It is important to avoid touching a boil with the fingers, because the infection can so easily spread to other areas. It is always best to take special care with boils on the face because of the danger of their spreading inward.

Bringing it to a head
Boils usually clear up by themselves, but you can help them to form a head—and ease the pain at the same time—by bathing the area with hot water or by applying a hot flannel or poultice.

Sties
Because a sty is right next to the eye, it is not possible to help it come to a head using the hot poultice method. An alternative is called hot-spoon bathing.

Heat a wooden spoon in boiling water. Flick off the water and wave the spoon around for a second to cool slightly. Then hold the rounded bowl of the spoon against the sty. When the spoon cools off, repeat the procedure. One other way to help the sty discharge its pus is to pull out the eyelash from the infected follicle. This can be painful and must be done very carefully.

Squeezing boils
Although small boils can be gently squeezed without much danger, it is wise to leave them alone. Large or painful boils must certainly never be squeezed, nor should you squeeze carbuncles or any boils, large or small, that are located between the eye and nose.

Once a boil has burst and the pus begins to drain, a dry dressing should be applied daily. This prevents the bacteria in the pus from spreading the infection and also prevents clothes from rubbing against the boil, which will slow the healing and may introduce further infection.

Medical attention
In rare circumstances when the pus remains trapped, a doctor may decide to lance a boil. If the inflammation appears to be spreading or a carbuncle is forming, he or she may prescribe a course of antibiotics.

A series of recurring boils can occasionally be a sign of a condition such as diabetes or another illness. Anyone suffering from recurring boils should be sure to seek medical advice in order to eliminate these possibilities.

Medical attention should also be sought if, in addition to one or more boils, there is a high temperature or general feeling of illness. The very young or very old should also consult a doctor as soon as possible if they develop a boil, as boils can be more serious in these age groups.

Carbuncles
Carbuncles (two or more boils occurring next to each other) are more serious than single boils, and they must receive medical attention from a doctor. Plenty of rest is necessary in their treatment, especially in the elderly, for carbuncles can make a person feel ill.

Avoiding boils

Do
- keep fit and healthy
- wash regularly, especially in places where there is rubbing, such as the buttocks and neck
- powder neck and buttocks with talc to reduce friction and sweat formation

Don't
- allow yourself to get run-down or anemic
- wash with dirty washcloths
- wear nylon underwear or tight collars if you are prone to boils

Treating boils

Do
- dress a draining boil daily
- get advice from a doctor if you have a series of boils, a general illness, or a high temperature
- take care with boils on the face

Don't
- pick at boils or you will spread the infection
- squeeze a boil before the head has formed
- squeeze a carbuncle or a large or painful boil
- attempt to sterilize your skin with household disinfectant. It does not work and can be dangerous

---

Bones

Bones are light, extremely strong, and joined so that the human body is highly mobile. There are few serious bone diseases, and these are usually treatable.

Most people think of bones simply as a stiffening framework deep inside the body that helps to keep us upright. This is basically true, but the reason why bones exist is somewhat different.

Bones are, in fact, a reminder of the fight for survival that all animals faced in the earliest stage of life on Earth. They were protection from damage or attack, and almost all successful primitive land creatures carried their bones outside the body—like the bony armor-plating commonly called a shell. Only later did some groups of animals develop so that their shells grew partially, then completely, inside the body, forming bones as we know them.

In humans, of course, bones reach the highest form of development, each of the hundreds of different bones in the body being joined to the next to create a fantastically strong, yet agile, framework: the skeleton.

The need for bones

The primitive function of bones as armor-plating is still obvious today in certain parts of the human body. One only needs to think of the skull, which forms a complete protective case around the brain, or

Different types of bones

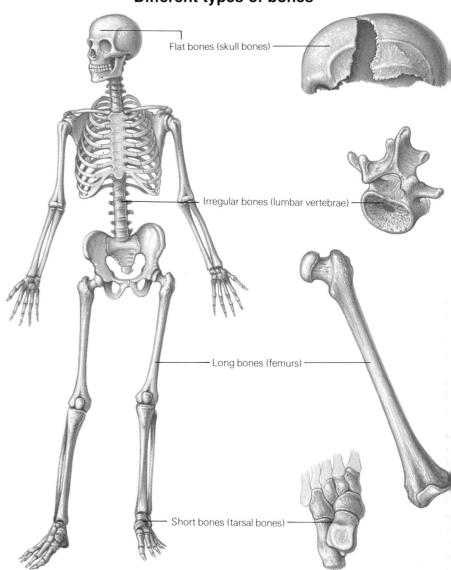

Flat bones (skull bones)

Irregular bones (lumbar vertebrae)

Long bones (femurs)

Short bones (tarsal bones)

Cross section of a long bone

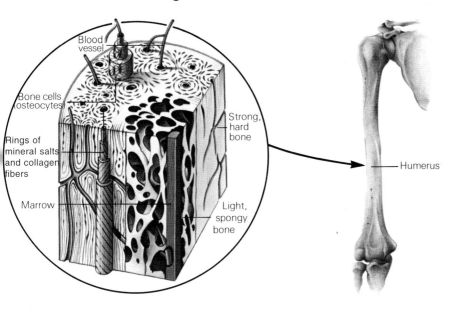

- Blood vessel
- Bone cells (osteocytes)
- Rings of mineral salts and collagen fibers
- Marrow
- Strong, hard bone
- Light, spongy bone
- Humerus

the ribs, which do the same thing for the heart and lungs.

Bones also, of course, provide the support that keeps the many components of the body together and upright. When the body thinks support is no longer needed—such as in the prolonged weightlessness of space flight, or just the experience of rest in bed—the bones will lose their strength and will break easily if put under strain.

Another vital, but not quite so obvious, use of bones is as girders to which muscles may be attached. Muscles provide the power by which the various limbs and body parts are moved, and this is done in the first place by moving the bones relative to each other.

The insides of bones are hollow, and the body, with great economy of space, uses these cavities for the manufacture of blood cells. They also store another vital substance for the body—calcium.

The structure of bones

Like everything else in the body, bones are made up of cells. They are of a type that creates what is technically called a fibrous tissue framework, a relatively soft and pliable material, osteroid.

The osteroid becomes a base for the deposition of calcium and phosphorus compounds that give strength and rigidity to bone.

The growth of bones

When bones begin growing, they are solid throughout. Only at a secondary stage do they start to develop hollow centers. Hollowing out a tube of material reduces its strength only very slightly, while very much reducing its weight.

Nature takes full advantage of this basic structural law in the design of bones. The hollow centers are filled with a soft substance, called marrow, where the blood cells are manufactured.

Bones start forming in a human baby during the first month of pregnancy, but just like the skeletons of primitive creatures, they are at this stage made of cartilage, a soft material with a rubbery flexibility. As the baby grows, this cartilage frame is replaced by fibrous tissue with little or none of the hardening agent. Hardening of the bones is a gradual process that takes place throughout childhood and is only completed by the end of puberty.

Keeping in shape

Another important and remarkable feature of bones is their ability to grow into the right shape. This is especially important for the long bones that support the limbs. These are wider at each end than in the middle, and this provides extra solidity at the joint where it is most needed. This shaping, which is technically known as modeling, is specially engineered during growth and goes on all the time afterward.

Different shapes and sizes

There are several different types of bone, designed to perform in varying ways. Long bones, forming the limbs, are simply cylinders of hard bone with the soft, spongy marrow interior.

Short bones, for example, those found at the wrist and ankle, have basically the same form as long bones but are more squat to allow a variety of movements without any consequent loss of strength.

Flat bones consist of a sandwich of hard bone with a spongy layer in between. They provide either protection (as in the skull, to protect the vulnerable brain) or a large area for attaching muscles (as in the shoulder blades).

The final bone type, irregular bones, comes in several different shapes, designed specifically for the job they do. The bones of the spine, for example, are box-shaped to give strength and plenty of space inside the marrow. And the bones that make up the structure of the face are hollowed out into air-filled cavities to create extra lightness.

The joints

Bones have to be joined securely to one another, but some must be able to move very extensively in relation to each other. The way nature solves this problem is with two types of joint—ball-and-socket type and hinge type.

The ends of the bones are lined with a pad of soft cartilage so that in movement and weight-bearing they do not damage each other. The joint is also lubricated by specially produced fluids. Tying the whole structure together are tough thongs called ligaments.

This X ray shows a clear fracture of the tibia (shinbone), the larger of the two bones in the lower leg.

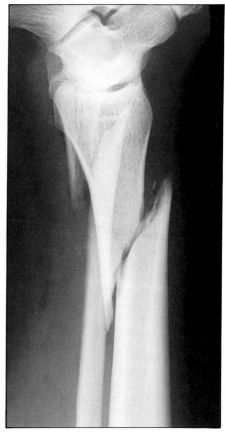

Derek Ellis

Q I saw an X ray of my ten-year-old son's arm, and there seemed to be lots of breaks in it. Yet the doctor said that the bone was not broken. Can this be true?

A The breaks you saw were gaps between the growing points of the long bones. They join together after puberty, but in a ten-year-old they can give quite a confusing picture.

Q The doctor says my brother has osteomyelitis. How did he catch it, and is it serious?

A Osteomyelitis is a bone infection. It seems to occur in an area where there has been a previous injury—perhaps a break. Stray bacteria in the bloodstream from a cut or chest infection then multiply in this area, where the bone's natural defenses against infection have been reduced. It can almost always be cured.

Q Why do bones in the elderly break so easily?

A With increasing age bones often have a tendency to become less solid and thus more brittle; this is called osteoporosis. The bones get generally thinner and weaker with a loss of both mineral and fibrous tissue components. The condition can be improved by treatment. Other bone diseases are common in the elderly and predispose them to fractures. They include Paget's disease and cancer. Patients on long-term steroid therapy may also develop thinner bones.

Q The skeleton seems to be a remarkable piece of engineering, very light but also strong and maneuverable. So why do humans suffer so much from backache?

A When humans began walking on two legs instead of four, we used the same skeleton that had been evolved for four-legged animals. Unfortunately we didn't develop any further. Thus while we are well adapted horizontally, vertical postures create strain at the center of gravity situated at the bottom of the back, causing pain.

Self-maintenance

Like many other parts of the body, bones have the extraordinary capacity to maintain themselves if infected or damaged. The most obvious example of this is the ability to repair themselves when broken—even completely in two.

People often find it hard to imagine how this can happen. The key to it in the first place is the fact that when a bone breaks, blood vessels running through the bone automatically break too. Quite a large blood loss results (and needs to be replaced in many cases), but it is this blood lying around the area of the break that creates the scaffolding for the repair of the break by clotting (i.e., hardening) into a solid mass.

Next, cells from the broken ends of the bone spread into the clotted area and lay down fibrous tissue. This unites the two broken ends, but before the joint is really complete, the hardening process must take place.

The finished joint is actually rather large and unwieldy, forming a mass of new bone around the place of the break. But later on the bone's ability to shape itself remodels the area into the original, smooth shape.

This takes place over a period of years after the break is completely mended and the limb once again in use, so that eventually the place of the break—doctors call it a fracture—is unrecognizable from original, smooth bone, except by X rays.

Congenital diseases

Congenital diseases of bone are fortunately rare. They are severely crippling and in some cases fatal. Some of these conditions are due to a lack of enzymes needed for formation of the ground substance, with resultant buildup of the chemicals that should be processed by these enzymes. In other cases ground substance formation is defective for unknown reasons. The end result is increased fragility of the skeleton, with a tendency toward numerous fractures and, in some cases, dwarfism and marked skeletal deformities.

Chemical problems

Bone is undergoing constant resorption and reformation. This process is influenced by numerous hormones and vitamins. Softening of the bone, or osteomalacia, results when these substances are present in abnormal amounts.

The hormone PTH is made by the parathyroid glands and is concerned with maintenance of normal calcium levels in the blood. Bones are the reservoir for the body's calcium stores, and bone is destroyed when more calcium is needed than is supplied by the diet. This may

Repair of a fractured bone

A

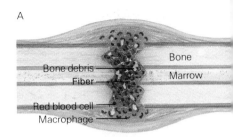

The site of the break is full of blood—which clots through the action of red cells, platelets, and fiber—and bone debris, which is removed by macrophages (large white blood cells). Surrounding bone produces cells that form the swollen or callus areas, one on either side of the break, and that will create new bone.

B

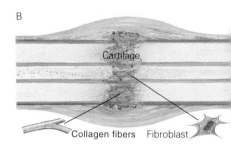

Fibroblasts (fibrous tissue cells) from intact bone produce collagen fibers, which help to make connective tissue.

C

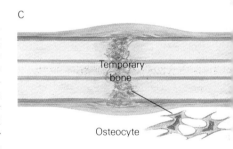

Cartilage is replaced and made more rigid by osteocytes (bone-producing cells); this creates temporary bone at the site of the fracture.

D

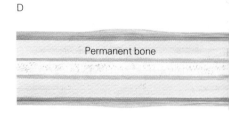

Temporary bone is replaced by permanent bone, and callus is reabsorbed. The total process generally takes a minimum of four to six weeks.

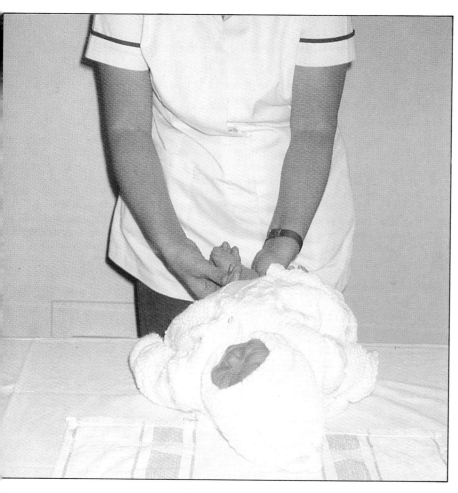

Even very young infants may need physiotherapy. Here the physiotherapist is demonstrating to this child's mother the technique of stretching a mild clubfoot.

happen in a number of ways. Sometimes a tumor forms in one of the glands, which then produces too much hormone, even though the calcium level is normal. More frequently the glands enlarge as a result of a persistently low blood-calcium level due to disease in other parts of the body. Calcium absorption is impaired in chronic kidney disease, severe intestinal malabsorption, and after resection of a large portion of the stomach.

All of these factors can cause the parathyroids to enlarge and produce excess hormone that will demineralize and weaken the bone. This condition can be treated by removing the excess parathyroid tissue.

Deficiency of essential vitamins

Vitamin D deficiency by itself can produce the same effect. The disease that it causes, called rickets (see Rickets), was once very widespread, but today it has been virtually eliminated by added vitamin D supplements in food.

Vitamin C deficiency also weakens bones by impairing production of ground substance, but this condition—called scurvy—is also practically unknown in the West today. Vitamin A deficiency or excess also had adverse effects on bone

formation in the past. And finally, a diet that is deficient in calcium (see Calcium) itself will produce the same adverse effects as a vitamin D deficiency.

Infections

Infections of bone are called osteomyelitis. They may result from direct invasion of the bone by external trauma or may be spread via the blood from another site of infection in the body. The most frequently involved organisms are *Staphylococcus aureus* and gram-negative bacilli.

Tuberculous osteomyelitis was once a common disease, but improved antitubercular drugs have largely eliminated it. Osteomyelitis is a serious and debilitating disease, but it can now almost always be cured by treatment involving large doses of antibiotics.

Bone tumors

The most common primary malignant tumor of bone is osteogenic sarcoma, which predominantly affects people

under 30 years of age. Once invariably fatal, today the tumor can frequently be cured by using combined treatments of X ray, surgery, and chemotherapy. The affected limb may be salvaged by replacement grafts.

Bone, because of its rich blood supply, is frequently invaded by tumors from other body sites, such as breast, prostate, and lung. Although they are usually not curable, these tumors can be controlled by hormone therapy, chemotherapy, and X-ray treatment in varying combinations, giving the patient a period of reasonable comfort and activity.

Osteoporosis

Osteoporosis (see Osteoporosis) is a poorly understood disease that affects the elderly, especially women, and produces thinning and brittleness of the bones. It probably has multiple causes, including diminished bone formation, accelerated bone destruction, calcium deficiency, and declining levels of the hormone estrogen in the post-menopausal woman.

It causes almost three-quarters of the fractures in women over 45, and it is likely to become an even greater problem as the elderly population increases. There is no specific treatment, but exercise and calcium and estrogen supplements may help. The decreased physical activity of old age also contributes to bone loss.

Immobilization osteoporosis is a thinning of bone caused by lack of use. Long familiar as a result of prolonged rest in bed, paralysis, or plaster cast immobilization for fractures, it is now becoming a problem in space exploration, due to the prolonged period of weightlessness experienced in orbiting flights. The cause is not known, but it may be due to abnormal sensitivity of the immobilized part to thyroid and parathyroid hormones.

Paget's disease

Paget's disease is characterized by local acceleration of bone resorption and deposition, producing markedly disordered growth. It usually involves multiple areas of the skeleton (especially the skull, pelvis, and leg bones) and predisposes the sufferer to the development of malignant tumors (osteogenic sarcoma).

The future

Considering how extensive and how complicated the human skeleton is, with its complex network of surrounding cartilage and tendons, it is prone to comparatively few problems—and today, most bone conditions are curable, or at least, controllable. Therefore, bone diseases need not be dreaded in the same way that they were before the advent of modern medical treatments.

Botulism

Botulism is a virulent form of food poisoning. Indeed the toxin is so potent that just half a pound (225 grams) would kill everyone in the world. Fortunately it is very rare, and commonsense cooking can prevent it.

Q I make my own jams and have heard that home preserving can cause botulism. Am I putting my family at risk by doing this?

A No, because the botulism poison is destroyed by the acidity of fruit. However, it can flourish in preserved meats if they are not canned properly. Though sugar is added to many preserves to eliminate their acid taste, it does not alter their chemical acidity, so there is still no risk.

Q Should I avoid the dented cans of food you sometimes see in the supermarket?

A These cans present problems with bacterial poisoning of other types, but there is no risk of botulism poisoning. It is therefore wise to choose undented cans.

Q Should I use a pressure cooker for canned vegetables to play it safe?

A Commercial canners plan their sterilization programs to kill botulism spores. If you can vegetables at home, pressure cooking is more advisable to be on the safe side.

Q Is there only one type of botulism?

A No, there are five distinct types of botulism toxin, and each is produced by a specific strain of bacteria. An antitoxin has been produced for each one, but even with treatment, mortality is still about 30 percent. This is why preventing the problem in the first place is so important.

Q I read that botulism can affect animals. How does this come about?

A Most animals are sensitive to the effects of botulism toxin, though sensitivity varies. For example, ducks are very sensitive to type E toxin, which has little effect on humans. An outbreak occurred in London parks during the 1976 drought, and water levels fell so low that the ducks became infected from the mud at the bottom of the pond.

Botulism is one of the rarest forms of food poisoning, but it is also one of the most deadly. It is caused by the bacterium *Clostridium botulinum* growing in the food, which produces a deadly poison called botulinum toxin. This organism is only able to grow well (and produce poison) in the complete absence of oxygen.

When unable to grow, it forms bacterial seeds called spores, which survive anywhere. If they get into food, they will survive the sort of boiling that eliminates other bacteria, and they can only be killed by cooking in a pressure cooker at 250°F (120°C) for at least 15 minutes.

Conditions for growth

However, they are also harmless unless they grow, so there are no dangers from such contamination except in foods processed so that air is excluded.

This means canned and bottled foods or foods sealed in airtight packs, or preserved meats, such as sausages. Of course bacteria do not grow if food is frozen, but once raised to room temperature any spore will start to germinate, and so such food must be eaten within a few days.

Canned foods should be sterilized by pressure cooking after the canning process, and unless the canning process is inadequate, the food is safe. Foods such as patés cannot be treated in this way, and great care must be taken to insure that such food is eaten within a day or two after purchase.

Unlike the spore, the growing *Clostridium* is easily destroyed, but unfortunately its poison is not. It will survive boiling for up to five minutes.

Eliminating the risks

Botulism is extremely rare. Commercial food processors are well aware of the risks, and they design their food preservation procedures to prevent it. Outbreaks have almost always been associated with home-preserved foods—for example, potted meats or vegetables.

The poison in action

The symptoms of botulism poisoning develop within two hours of eating the affected food. The toxin affects the brain and nervous system, making a person feel dizzy. They may have double vision, headaches, and progressive paralysis. Once the ability to breathe is lost, he or she dies. Accompanying symptoms may include nausea, vomiting, and diarrhea.

A bacterium called Clostridium botulinum *(inset) causes botulism. It does not affect bottled fruits but can affect paté.*

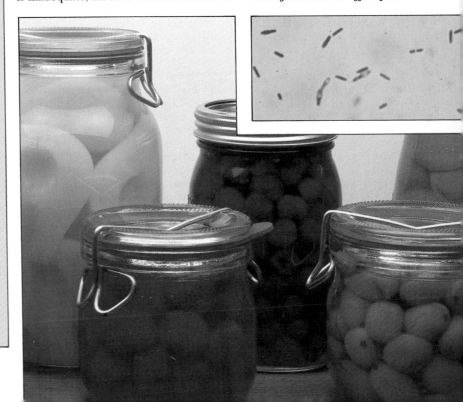

Brain

The human brain is more sophisticated than the largest computer—yet it fits neatly inside the skull. With its many millions of cells, it directs and monitors all our activities, even when we are asleep or unconscious.

Q Sometimes when I smell something that I haven't smelled for a long time, old memories come flooding back. How does this happen?

A The connections in the brain for the sense of smell are closely linked with the circuits of the limbic system, which deals with emotions. Smells can thus take on clear emotional significance, whether pleasant or unpleasant. Because events associated with strong emotions are often well stored in memory, the smell itself can bring them back.

Q My friend says he's more intelligent than me because his head is larger. Is there any truth in this?

A Probably not. Intelligence is more to do with what you do with your brain than how much you have. Some people's brains are probably better at organizing their perceptions, relating them to memories, and forming plans of action on the basis of all this information. The emotional level that the brain is operating at is also very important. Too little emotion deprives the brain of essential psychological energy, while too much causes poor concentration.

Your personality—especially the way that you react to problems and cope with your emotions—is a big factor in determining how intelligent you become.

Q My memory is dreadful. Is there anything I can do to improve it?

A It is not your memory that needs improving, it is the way you try to remember things. In order to make certain that something is firmly stored, it must be presented to the brain in a way that arouses the most associations, or links, with other knowledge that you have already stored there. For example, a written description of directions to a place is rather cumbersome to remember—a map or drawing is much easier and stays fixed in the mind for a longer time. And if the map is humorous, the memory will be even stronger, because the emotions are involved.

The brain is at the center of the complex network of nerves that runs through the body, and together with the spinal cord (see Spinal cord), it makes up what is known as the central nervous system.

Lines of communication

The central nervous system controls the whole body by means of messages that are continually passing up and down its nerve pathways. All the information a person receives about his or her surroundings comes from the five senses—sight, hearing, touch, smell, and taste. The nerves carrying this sensory information up to the brain are called sensory nerves. Once the brain makes a decision, it sends its instructions for action down other nerve cells called motor nerves.

Short circuit

All nerve impulses going to and from the brain have to go up or down the spinal cord. But now and then, for example, if a person touches a flame, such speedy action is needed that there is no time for the message to go all the way to the brain. The message goes only as far as the spinal cord, which processes the message and responds to it on a relatively simple level. The result is called a reflex.

When a doctor taps a patient's knee and makes it jerk, he or she is looking for possible damage to the spinal cord by testing how fast the reflexes are. Other examples of reflexes are blinking, reactions to pain, and sexual responses.

Inside the skull

All the messages flashing to and from the brain are transmitted by minute electrical impulses. They travel through special nerve tissue cells called neurons. The electrical activity in the brain creates waves that can be picked up on a machine called an electroencephalogram, or EEG, and studied for abnormal or unusual patterns.

Major divisions of the brain

The brain consists of the brain stem, the cerebellum, and the cerebrum, which has four lobes. Body activities (see examples in cerebrum) are controlled by specific areas within the brain.

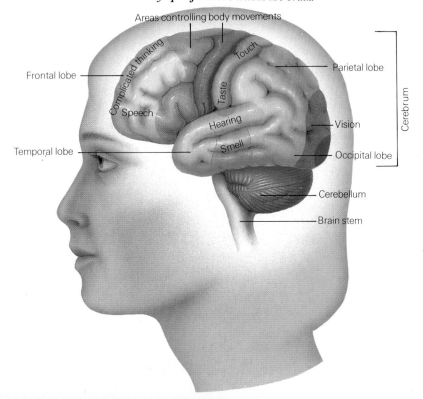

Areas controlling body movements

Complicated thinking

Touch

Frontal lobe

Taste

Parietal lobe

Speech

Hearing

Vision

Cerebrum

Temporal lobe

Smell

Occipital lobe

Cerebellum

Brain stem

Mike Courtney

BRAIN

The brain cells form a mass of soft, jellylike tissue, surrounded by three layers of protective membrane called the meninges and some fluid called cerebrospinal fluid. Four arteries in the neck supply the brain with blood, without which it cannot survive.

Mapping the brain

Basically the brain can be divided into three different regions: hindbrain, midbrain, and forebrain. Each of these is divided into separate areas responsible for quite distinct functions, all intricately connected to other parts of the brain.

Balance and coordination

The largest structure in the hindbrain is the cerebellum. This is the area that is in charge of balance and coordination, and it works very closely with the organs of balance in the inner ear.

Early origins

Also part of the hindbrain is the brain stem, which links the brain with the

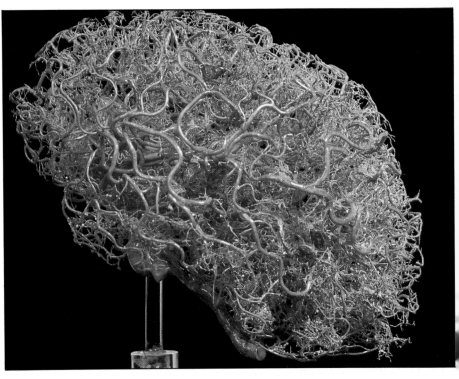

This resin cast shows the vital network of vessels that supply blood to the brain. Brain cells die within a few minutes if starved of oxygenated blood.

Internal structures of the brain

This cross section highlights the major structures of the brain. The limbic system (inset), located within the thalamus, is chiefly concerned with memory, learning, and emotions.

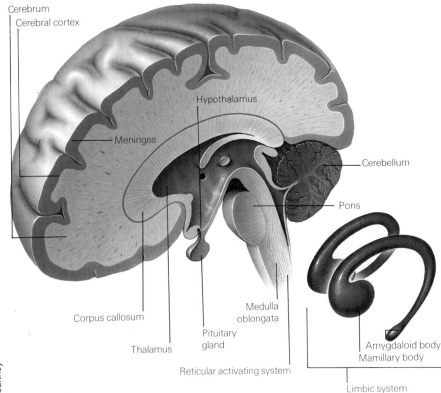

Cerebrum
Cerebral cortex
Hypothalamus
Meninges
Cerebellum
Pons
Corpus callosum
Medulla oblongata
Thalamus
Pituitary gland
Amygdaloid body
Mamillary body
Reticular activating system
Limbic system

Mike Courtney

spinal cord. This is the part of the brain that was first to evolve in primitive human beings. It is here in the brain stem that all incoming and outgoing messages come together and cross over, for the left side of the body is governed by the right-hand side of the brain, and right side of the body by the left-hand side of the brain.

The various structures in the brain stem, including those called the medulla, pons, and reticular-activating system, are in charge of life itself—for they control heart rate, blood pressure, swallowing, coughing, hiccuping, vomiting, breathing, and consciousness.

Brain censor and other structures

One of the brain's most crucial functions is controlling the level of consciousness. A mechanism in the brain stem's reticular-activating system sifts through the mass of incoming information and decides which is important enough to alert the brain to. It does this by controlling the amount of electrical activity that each part of the brain receives.

In turn the reticular-activating system is affected by the brain's decisions. It is this interplay that determines alertness and consciousness.

Just beyond the brain stem, in the midbrain, is an area devoted to controlling eye movements and pupil size. Beyond this the forebrain begins. Here the

Proportions of the cortex devoted to sensory and motor activities

The cortex (surface of the cerebrum) has one area that is just concerned with receiving sensory or incoming information (left), and another area that deals with

outgoing or motor information (right). The amount of cortex devoted to receiving or giving information depends on the specific part of the body concerned. For instance, a

large part of the sensory cortex is given to the lips because they are very sensitive; a large part of the motor cortex is related to sending out information to the hands.

Incoming information—sensory

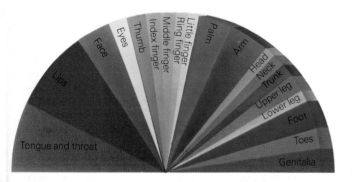

Outgoing information—motor

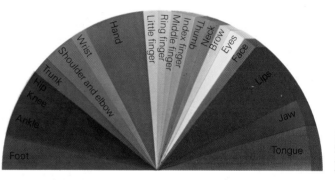

Aziz Khan

thalamus is located, acting as a sort of relay station for incoming information.

Just below the thalamus is the hypothalamus. This is involved in such bodily functions as hunger and thirst, body temperature, sex, and sleep, and it works closely with the pituitary gland.

Deep-seated emotions
Nearby is another important system: the limbic system, made up of a number of structures including the hippocampus, amygdala, and septum pelucidum. This is the second most primitive part of the brain and is concerned with deep-seated emotions like rage, excitement, fear, sexual interest, pleasure, and even sociability.

The limbic system is closely connected with the smell centers of the brain, and there are also rich connections with areas involved with the other senses, behavior, and the organization of memories.

In addition to information from our sense organs, we also receive messages from our internal organs, and these are relayed to the decision-making part of the brain by the limbic system. This accounts for the fact that these particular sensations are usually tinged with emotion—and that emotions can affect digestion.

Divided in two
The largest part of the brain is the cerebrum, located in the forebrain. It is divided right down the middle into two halves called hemispheres, which are joined at the bottom by a thick bundle of nerve fibers called the corpus callosum. Although the two hemispheres are mirror images of each other, they have completely different functions and work together through the corpus callosum.

Higher processes
The cerebrum is more developed in humans than in any other animal and is essential to thought, memory, consciousness, and the higher mental processes. This is where the other parts of the brain send incoming messages for a decision.

Gray matter
The 0.1 in (3 mm) thick, wrinkled layer of gray matter folded over the outside of the cerebrum is called the cerebral cortex. This part of the brain has become so highly developed in humans that it has had to fold over and over in order to fit inside the skull. Unfolded, it would cover an area 30 times as large as when folded.

The four lobes
Among all the folds are certain very deep grooves that divide each of the two hemispheres of the cerebrum into four areas called lobes. The temporal lobes are involved with hearing and also with smell, the parietal lobes with touch, the occipital lobes with vision, and the frontal lobes with movement and complicated thinking.

Within each of these lobes, there are specific portions devoted to receiving the sensory messages from one area. The sense of touch, for example, has a tiny area in the parietal lobe devoted to nothing but sensation from the knee, and a large area for the thumb. This is why areas like the thumb are more sensitive than areas like the knee. And the same principle applies to the other sensory parts of the cerebrum, and to the motor, or movement, parts as well. Of course none of these areas of the brain can work by itself. Every instruction is, in effect, a joint

decision, resulting from the different areas comparing and pooling their information and then coordinating the resulting action.

Personality
Most human behavior consists of movements. In addition, an individual goes over possible behaviors in his or her head and uses language to think as well as act. This gives a sense of an individual's relationship to the outside world, which is felt as consciousness or personality.

While the entire brain takes part in this process, it is the frontal lobes that act as the organizing and coordinating areas. They are involved with directing a person's behavior in accordance with the plans they formulate; they also have the task of insuring that this behavior remains socially acceptable.

Memory and learning
No particular area of the brain stores all memories; in fact, memory is not a bank of information, but a process. When an electrical message passes through a brain cell, the cell changes physically. As a person learns something, new electrical pathways are set up that enable it to be remembered for a few minutes.

To remember something for a longer period of time, closer attention has to be paid to it, and it has to be gone-over many times. As a result a permanent physical change takes place in the brain cells themselves, which makes the memory literally a part of the person. Sometimes, however, a special trigger is needed to help recall a particular memory, while others seem to get buried so deep that, for all practical purposes, they are lost.

Brain damage and disease

Q I've read a lot in the news lately about brain death. Is it the same as ordinary death?

A Death is a process, not an event. The different cells in the body take different lengths of time to stop working when their blood supply is cut off. After the heart stops beating, it may take some hours before all the body's cells are dead.

Until recently death was said to have occurred when the heart had stopped and when there was no more breathing. But now medical therapy can prevent those two things from happening for long periods of time, even when there is no hope of consciousness being regained. So brain death is said to have occurred when all the signs show that the person will never regain consciousness.

It is very important, however, that strict guidelines are followed to make sure, in particular, that there are no drugs in the person's body that might confuse the issue.

Q My mother has recently had a stroke, and she cannot speak properly. Does this mean her mind is affected as well?

A Probably not. But the total effect of the working of the brain is what makes a mind. So large areas of damage can seem to affect a person's mind until the undamaged parts have taken over. With very severe strokes, there is so much damage that "internal" speech (which is one of the ways we think) is probably affected, and the mind is therefore altered.
In general a person's personality remains intact after a stroke.

Q I've heard that brain damage is less serious in children than in adults. How can this be?

A Any substantial brain damage is tragic. But children's brains are less rigid than adults', so other parts can more easily take over the function of a damaged section. For example, speech loss (or aphasia) after brain injury is usually not permanent in very young children. Even among preteen children, recovery is greater than in adults.

The skills and technology of modern medicine have completely changed attitudes toward brain damage and disorders and brought new hope to those afflicted.

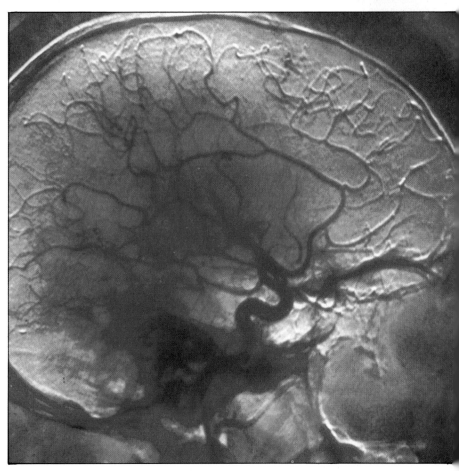

The brain arteries have been injected with a fluid to show up on the X ray.

The brain is made up of millions of highly complicated nerve cells and connections that the eye cannot see. Many parts of the brain are still completely uncharted. Yet today, when something goes wrong, specialists know enough about the brain to work out what may be wrong—usually by a process of elimination, discarding the most unlikely problems. They then perform tests, generally with electronic machinery such as the computerized tomography (CT) scan (which gives an X-ray picture of sections of the brain), to narrow down to a final diagnosis, on the basis of which treatment is arranged.

Positive attitudes
It is very important for those with friends or family who suffer brain damage not to assume automatically that it is untreatable. It is easy to take this view, simply because brain damage sounds so serious—and in the past usually was—and also because brain damage usually causes very major and worrisome changes in the person concerned, such as loss of consciousness, paralysis, or loss of speech.

Remarkable recoveries
In fact, it is amazing how much recovery is possible. For example, after a severe blow to the head in a car crash, the patient may seem deeply unconscious; he or she may spend days without showing any sign of life. This can be the result of extensive, but temporary, paralysis of the neurons—the nerve cells—and if this is the case, large areas of the brain will eventually recover and will work normally again.

Spare parts
The brain also has what doctors call a large "reserve of function," which means that it contains spare areas that can take over the work damaged areas can no longer manage. Children, in particular,

can make astonishing recoveries from brain damage because their brains are not so rigidly organized as those of adults and the reserve areas can adapt more flexibly to what is required of them.

There is, however, a limit to the scope of recovery, and the key factor in this is how much damage has been done to the brain stem, the area through which all the brain's messages to the various regions of the body must pass. It also contains centers that keep up processes such as breathing and blood circulation. Without these, life soon slips away.

Life support
When a patient with severe brain damage is first brought in to the hospital, these vital functions may not be working. It is important to get the body functions working artificially (by means of special machinery called life support systems) until the brain recovers enough to take over again.

The introduction of these machines has meant the possibility of recovery where before there was no hope. But they also bring their problems. In a few days it may become clear that, however long support is given, recovery is impossible, because so much nerve tissue has been lost.

Such situations, of course, will be hard to accept, but occasionally people, including some doctors, have to face them. So the only realistic approach when someone is put on a life support machine is to remember that this does not mean there will be recovery, only that there is the possibility of it.

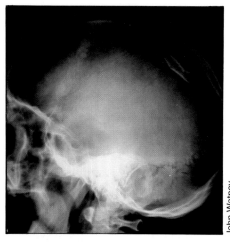

John Watney

Skull fractures can cause concussion and possibly brain injury. Here the fractures are visible at the top rear of the skull.

Principal brain diseases

Symptoms	Cause	Doctor's comments
Stroke Sudden weakness or loss of use and numbness of one side of body and/or loss of speech or other brain function	Blood vessel block (cerebral thrombosis) or rupture (with cerebral hemorrhage). Referred to as cerebrovascular accidents, or CVA	Usually affects older people. Disability always worse to start with, gradually improving to some degree
Multiple sclerosis Sudden blurring of vision, unsteadiness or loss of use of a limb. Patient tends to recover and then it returns. Slow increase in disability over years	Patchy inflammation of insulating material around nerves in brain and spinal cord. Basic cause remains unknown	Usually affects younger people. Wide variation in disability. Many will lead near normal lives for many years
Meningitis Headache, temperature, general illness. Stiff neck, dislike of light	Infection of brain's surrounding membranes, or meninges, by bacteria or viruses	If bacterial, needs antibiotics. Full recovery in most cases
Encephalitis Temperature, drowsiness, speech impairment, seizures	Virus infection of brain itself	Needs early treatment. May leave some damage
Dementia Loss of recent memory, easily confused, gradual loss of the intellect; eventual speech impairment and incontinence	Causes include: degeneration of cells of cerebral cortex, tumors, alcoholism, vitamin deficiency, and chronic infection	Mostly in older people. Some causes treatable, so must be investigated
Parkinson's disease Stiff muscles, difficulty starting movements, expressionless face, trembling fingers	Degeneration of cells deep in the base of the brain	Treatment with L-dopa helps to control symptoms
Epilepsy Tendency to have seizures, which may be major, with loss of consciousness and jerking of limbs; or minor, with odd sensations and short lapses of consciousness; or confined to jerking of limb	Electrical storm in brain due to abnormal excitability of some of the neurons. May come on later in life and be caused by tumors or brain injury	Treatment will control seizures. May need special tests to establish cause

Blows to the head
One of the most common head injuries is caused by some sort of blow. The effect of a blow to the head is determined by the severity and the location, as well as the angle of the blow. Even slight blows can sometimes cause concussion, the medical name for the loss of consciousness caused by such an injury. Concussion itself is the mildest form of brain injury, and it may cause no real permanent damage. If the blow is severe, there may be headaches, giddiness, and lowered concentration for some weeks after.

Sometimes the brain may actually be bruised as a result of a blow. In this case there will be some permanent damage to the nerve cells and fibers, but how this affects the person depends on the amount of bruising.

Internal bleeding from an injury
If a blow is severe, blood vessels in the brain or in the protective membranes around it can be torn. This causes bleeding inside the brain called a brain hemorrhage (see Hemorrhage). If a blood clot forms just under or just outside the outer membrane, it will put pressure upon the brain, and surgery is often necessary to remove the clot.

Sometimes the bleeding occurs as a slow ooze, which exerts an increasing pressure on the brain over a number of days. This can cause symptoms like headaches, nausea, and drowsiness to occur long after the injury. If the clot that forms is large, surgery may be necessary.

Loss of memory
Often a person who has had a concussion will not remember what took place just before the injury. This is a result of there not having been time after the injury for the memory to process the events.

Q What do people mean when they say that a boxer is punch-drunk?

A Some of the repeated head blows that a boxer suffers are enough to cause tiny hemorrhages, or bleeding, in various parts of the brain. Each blow is not enough in itself to cause trouble, but over the years the damage mounts up.

There is slurring of speech and unsteadiness on the feet due to damage, especially to the cerebellum, which controls balance and coordination. In addition the boxer's mind may become a little less sharp, with some confusion and loss of memory. This is caused by damage to the cerebral cortex, which controls thinking. All this makes the boxer appear drunk.

Q My sister has just had a baby, and they had to give it some oxygen after the birth. Can this cause brain damage?

A No, it can't. It is very important to make sure that babies have enough oxygen in their blood, ᴇspecially after a difficult birth, to prevent brain damage. However, careful measurement of the amount of oxygen being given must be made, because very high concentrations can cause damage to a baby's eyes and to the cells lining the air passages.

Q I've heard that watching TV can cause epileptic seizures. Is this true?

A Yes—but only in some people and with some televisions. In a small number of people already prone to them, seizures can be brought on by flickering lights. Like the strobe lights found at discos, some televisions flicker at just the right rate to bring on seizures. This does not mean that a person with epilepsy cannot watch television, since it has no effect on most epileptics.

Q Could I damage my child's brain by not giving her enough fish in her diet?

A No. This myth probably arose because fish was once a cheap source of protein important to the growth of a child's brain.

Tests for disorders

Procedure	Purpose	Doctor's comments
Lumbar puncture Removal of some cerebrospinal fluid from base of spine	To detect infection, inflammation, or bleeding in or around brain	Nowadays only slightly uncomfortable, done under local anesthetic
EEG (electroencephalogram) Recording of electrical activity of brain from electrodes on scalp	To detect abnormal electrical discharge in investigation of blackouts or fits	Painless
CT scan X-ray scan of brain linked to computer, showing horizontal layers of brain	To detect tumors, abscesses, and areas of brain damage	Painless and harmless. May need injection of dye into vein to make abnormality more visible
MRI (Magnetic Resonance Imaging) scan Shows cross sections of the brain	To detect tumors, abscesses, and areas of brain damage	No radiation
Cerebral arteriogram Direct injection of arteries with fluid that shows up on X ray	To detect abnormalities or blocks in arteries	Usually done under general anesthetic

Following a bad injury to the head, a person may have difficulty concentrating after regaining consciousness. As a result, memories will not be laid down properly in the brain, even though the person may appear to have recovered. How long the condition lasts will depend on the severity of the injury.

A blow that is hard enough to fracture or break the skull will usually also cause concussion. The fracture itself causes little trouble unless the broken part of the skull is pushed inward, tearing the brain tissue and causing bleeding.

Penetrating injuries
An injury to the head from falling onto a sharp object like a pencil, or other items that actually penetrate the skull, exposes the surface of the brain to infection. In addition the object itself may carry infection into the brain. The amount of damage that is done in any injury of this type depends on where the object enters.

Bullet wounds to the head carry these risks and additional dangers as well. Their explosive entry into the skull sends shock waves through the brain that can disrupt very distant nerve cells and also cause tearing of the blood vessels.

Brain damage at birth
If, during birth, the blood supply to a baby's brain is inadequate for some reason, some of his or her brain cells will die. If a lot of cells are damaged, a condition called cerebral palsy results. Similar brain damage can occur after birth if an infant is starved of oxygen because of a lung disorder. The term *spastic* used to be used to describe these children because of the stiffness of the muscles, especially in the legs, that is caused by such brain damage.

The number of limbs affected and the severity of the condition varies from child to child. The level of intelligence also varies—some children with cerebral palsy may be mentally retarded, while others are of normal or high intelligence.

Abnormal growths
Abnormal growths in the tissue of the brain are called brain tumors. The most common cause is cancer somewhere else in the body, in which case the growth is called a secondary tumor.

Like other tumors, brain tumors can be either malignant (cancerous) or benign (noncancerous). Malignant tumors are those that grow quickly and tend to invade the surrounding tissues. Benign tumors do not invade, but they can create trouble as they grow, pushing against the rest of the brain and causing it to distort.

Treatment of growths
Once a tumor has been detected, it is essential to find out whether it is malignant or benign. An operation called a biopsy may be necessary in order to obtain a piece of the lump for examination under the microscope, to determine the nature of the cells.

Although there is often no possibility of removing secondary tumors, they can often be reduced in size by special X rays or drug treatment. Benign tumors and some slower-growing malignant tumors can often be removed surgically or be treated with drugs. The pressure of a growing tumor causes such symptoms as persistent headaches, nausea, and eventually drowsiness, leading to coma (very deep unconsciousness) if it is not discovered in time.

Symptoms of brain disease

In addition to the symptoms caused by the increasing pressure from a tumor, there are also other symptoms that indicate something is wrong. When a particular area of the brain becomes diseased, it will stop performing its own specific function properly.

A doctor will recognize these symptoms as a possible indication of some sort of disease in that area of the brain. A tumor is one possibility, but there are other diseases that can cause part of the brain to malfunction. Some of these are shown in the table on page 225.

The symptoms that appear as a result of a disease depend on the area of the brain affected. For example, symptoms of

Radioisotope scanners can be used to diagnose brain disease or damage.

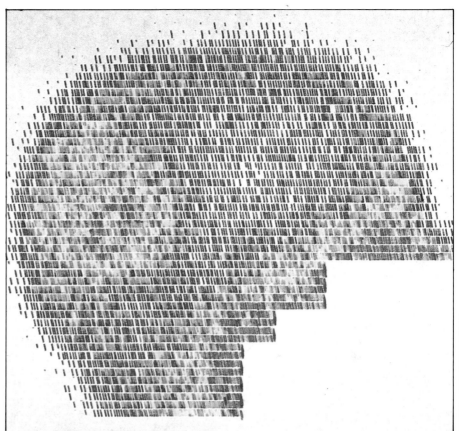

Daily Telegraph Colour Library

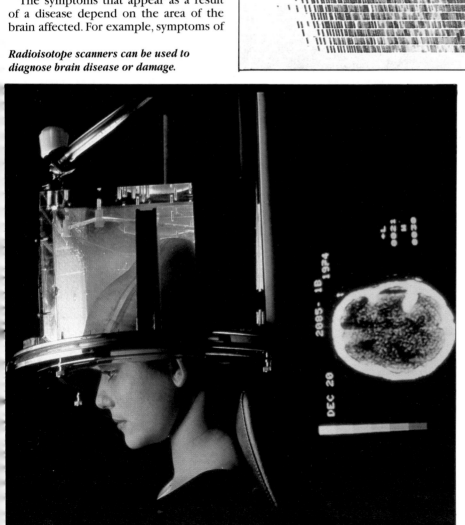

For this color scan a radioactive substance was injected into the brain. Some has drained out (right edge), but some has concentrated as a circular red area (left) of increased radioactivity, indicating a serious tumor.

disease in the left side of the brain might be hesitant or jumbled speech; difficulty in reading or writing; loss of feeling or vision; a general weakness on the right side; or a change in personality. These are all serious symptoms that need to be investigated by a doctor or specialist.

Symptoms of disease in the right side of the brain could include weakness, numbness, or visual loss on the left side of the body, or difficulty in dressing or in the person finding his or her way around.

Disease in the area of the thalamus, cerebellum, midbrain, or brain stem area can be indicated by a dramatic change in a person's mood; strange appetites; double vision; unsteadiness; severe giddiness; or a reduction in the ability to control breathing.

None of these symptoms is a definite indication of brain disease. A person who experiences any of these symptoms should see his or her family doctor, who will arrange the appropriate examinations and tests. It is always better to identify a disease in its early stages, as treatment will be more effective.

Brain surgery

Q My father just had a brain tumor removed. Can it grow again?

A If a tumor (either benign or malignant) is small and is sited in a suitable place, the surgeon will probably be able to remove all the tissues, thereby cutting down the risk of the tumor forming again. If a tumor is sited in an inaccessible place, the surgeon may not be able to remove the whole mass. The tumor may then grow again. However, a further operation can sometimes be done.

Q My six-year-old son has to have a brain operation. What are his chances of a complete recovery?

A This depends mainly on the exact site of the trouble. However, a child's brain is more amenable to surgery, because it is not fully developed and has a "plastic" quality. Since the young brain is more adaptable, recovery may be greater than in an adult, because the healthy areas of the child's brain take over some of the functioning of the damaged areas.

Q What are the latest advances in brain surgery?

A The most important advance is the development of microsurgery, using an operating microscope. Now the surgeon can do exceptionally delicate work on the brain.

Q My husband has a blood clot on the brain. Can it be removed by surgery?

A Depending on the site of the blood clot inside the skull, it may be possible to remove it by surgery. The major problem with all brain surgery is getting at the site of the trouble. Often it can only be reached by cutting through other parts of the brain. If it cannot be operated on, anticoagulants (drugs that lessen the likelihood of blood clotting) can be given. Alternative blood vessels may enlarge to provide an adequate supply to the affected part of the brain. All in all, chances of recovery are much better than they used to be.

Brain surgery has developed so rapidly in the last decade that complex operations are now available—and continuing research means that the outlook for patients is constantly improving.

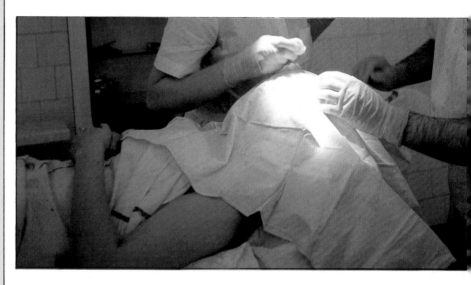

Today's delicate brain surgery can be used to treat a range of conditions that cause brain damage. Operations can be successfully performed where previously they would never have been attempted.

Blood clots
When a severe blow to the head occurs, the blood vessels in the meninges—the membranes covering the brain and the spinal cord—or in the brain itself, may be torn, and bleeding may occur. This is called a traumatic brain hemorrhage. A blood clot may form on the membrane lining the brain, putting pressure on the brain itself. Surgery is often required to remove the clot. Sometimes bleeding shows as a slow ooze, and pressure gradually builds up. This is called a chronic subdural hematoma. Here again surgery is called for. A general anesthetic is always given with brain surgery, and the patient is carefully monitored afterward. A few weeks' stay in the hospital is required.

A skull fracture can be caused, for example, by being hit over the head with a bottle or other heavy instrument. A blow hard enough to fracture the skull usually causes a concussion.

More serious is a depressed fracture, where the broken part of the bone has pushed into the underlying brain and torn its tissues. Surgery is needed.

A blood clot in the brain (thrombosis) occurs spontaneously. It builds up gradually and is often associated with high blood pressure. A clot can occur in any

Damage caused by a tumor, hemorrhage, or fracture may be repaired by surgery.

part of the brain. In some positions it may be possible to treat it by surgery; or anticoagulant drugs can be used.

Brain tumors
Tumors do not usually arise in the actual nerve cells but in the tissues that surround them—the neuroglia cells—or in the cells of the meninges. Sometimes tumors develop in the pituitary gland and press upward into the brain.

Like tumors elsewhere in the body, brain tumors can be either benign or malignant. Malignant tumors grow quickly and spread into the surrounding tissues. Benign tumors cause trouble because they grow slowly in the skull, pushing and distorting the brain. Depending on the location of the tumor, surgery may be possible. Where it is difficult to reach, radiotherapy or steroid drugs may be used to treat the condition.

Subarachnoid hemorrhage
Leaking may occur from a group of blood vessels near the base of the brain, with bleeding into the subarachnoid space, which will cause increasingly severe headaches or blackouts. This condition is due to a weakness in the vessels present since birth. The hemorrhage may happen spontaneously, or it may be triggered by an injury. An operation is necessary to tie up these blood vessels.

Breasts

Q My daughter is only 10, but her breasts are already quite well developed. Isn't this unusual at her age?

A No, perfectly normal—your daughter has just begun her sexual development a little earlier than average. It is important that you don't let her become embarrassed about her body at this time, when it is undergoing so many changes. It may help her self-confidence to take her out to choose some pretty light-support bras. Remember, too, that girls now mature a lot earlier than they did 40 years ago. Your daughter's friends will soon be catching up, if they haven't done so already.

Q I'm very embarrassed because my breasts are so large. Is there anything that can be done about them?

A If you are above average weight, losing some weight may help you to lose some of the excess fat in your breasts. In the meantime it might help to choose clothes that flatter your figure rather than overemphasizing your shape and to wear a well-fitting bra. Although doctors are reluctant to recommend surgery, if your breasts are still a problem, particularly if they are causing physical problems, breast tissue can be removed in an operation called a reduction mammoplasty.

Q My son is 15 and seems to be developing small breasts. He's very thin, so it's certainly not just fat. Is this serious? What can I do about it?

A Some boys do develop breastlike swellings during puberty that are not the result of being overweight but are due to the increased levels of sex hormones in their blood. The swellings, which may feel very tender and are a cause for extreme embarrassment in any boy, usually disappear on their own in 12 to 18 months. However, it might be wise to take him to see your doctor; this problem deserves medical attention in case it is a symptom of a more serious abnormality or needs surgical treatment.

The breasts are a very important part of a woman's body and of her self-image. Regular self-examination is essential to insure that all remains well.

Most people think of the budding of the breasts, which begins before the start of the menstrual periods, as the first sign that a girl is on the road from childhood into womanhood. In fact breasts appear in rudimentary form in both boys and girls long before birth and for a few days after birth, a baby of either sex may produce a few drops of colostrum, a nutritious fluid that appears before lactation (milk production) begins, from the nipples as a result of the action of the mother's hormones.

Development

At the start of sexual development, the pituitary gland at the base of the brain stimulates a girl's ovaries and they begin to release large amounts of the hormone estrogen. This hormone travels in the bloodstream to the breast area and triggers the enlargement of the nipples. It also encourages the growth of the channels, or lactiferous ducts, through which milk can be released when it is required to feed a baby, and the depositing of fat between and around them.

The completion of breast development, which takes about 18 months from the first appearance of small swellings on the chest, depends on another sex hormone, progesterone, which is produced monthly during the menstrual cycle. Under the influence of progesterone, the ends of the ducts swell out into lobes, each composed of many smaller lobes (called lobules) containing glands that lactate. Meanwhile the continued release of estrogen by the ovaries results in more fat developing between the lobules, until the breasts have fully developed.

The mature breast is roughly hemispherical in shape, with a tail-like extension toward the armpit. The slightly upward-pointing nipple contains 15 to 20 minute openings from the ducts. These are too small to be seen with the naked eye and are surrounded by a ring of darker tissue called the areola.

Aside from the tissues directly involved in the production and release of milk, each breast contains nerves and fibrous supporting tissue that gives it its firmness and shape. The nipple is particularly well supplied with nerves. These are important in breast-feeding, because it is their stimulation that causes the nipple to become erect.

What happens in pregnancy

Whether the breasts are large or small, they increase in size when a woman is

Structure of the breast

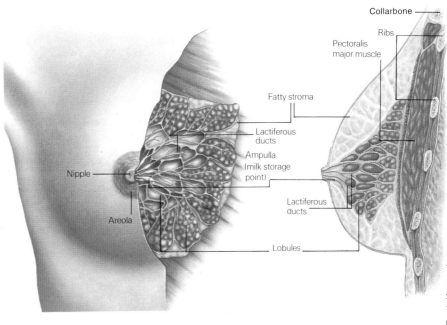

Collarbone

Ribs

Pectoralis major muscle

Fatty stroma

Lactiferous ducts

Ampulla (milk storage point)

Nipple

Lactiferous ducts

Areola

Lobules

Frank Kennard

229

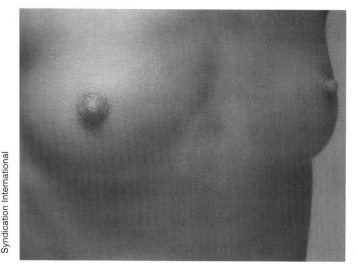
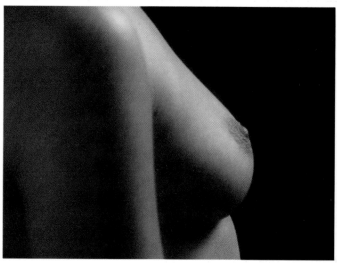

pregnant and may feel more tender than normal. During the course of pregnancy, the placenta makes enormous amounts of estrogen (see Estrogen), which, together with other hormones from the placenta and secretions from the thyroid and other glands, cause the ducts to grow in size and form more branches. At the same time the hormone progesterone, which is secreted by the placenta, stimulates the glandular tissue to enlarge.

Sacs, or alveoli, lined with true milk-producing cells are formed, and these produce the colostrum that flows into

At puberty large amounts of the hormone estrogen are released. This changes the adolescent breast (left) to that of the mature woman (right). This also promotes growth of milk ducts and deposits of fat, which give the breast its shape.

the ducts and out through the nipples even before birth. Large amounts of fat are also deposited in the breasts during pregnancy, so that the total breast weight increases by about 2 lb (1 kg). Through the effects of hormones, the areola around the nipple becomes darker.

Although they stimulate breast enlargement during pregnancy, the hormones estrogen and progesterone, created by the placenta, are thought to suppress the secretion of milk until after the baby is born. But immediately following birth—and the loss of the placenta and its hormones—the pituitary gland in the brain begins to make the hormone prolactin, which stimulates the milk-producing cells. For the first two or three days the cells secrete colostrum—the thin, yellowish fluid that contains the protein, minerals, and nutrients necessary for the baby. They then release true milk.

Breast care
Because the breasts contain no muscle, they are naturally likely to sag with age. The fibrous tissue within them becomes less elastic, and the heavier the breasts, the more likely this is to happen. This does not mean that it is essential to wear a bra, particularly if the breasts are naturally small, but many women find it more comfortable to have their breasts supported, if only lightly.

Another much more important part of routine breast care for all women over the age of 20, is to get into the habit of making a thorough examination of each breast. This examination should be done immediately after the menstrual period, when the breasts are smallest, or for women past menopause, at monthly intervals. What you must look for are any abnormal lumps or swellings that may need medical investigation.

It is recommended that all women over the age of 50 have regular breast examinations performed by a doctor, and a mammogram (an X-ray examination of the breasts) on a yearly basis. Whether this should be extended to include women between the ages of 40 and 50 remains a controversial issue.

Breast problems

Symptoms	Possible causes	Action
Fullness and discomfort	Premenstrual changes, effects of the Pill, breast development at puberty	Try taking extra vitamin B, but if symptoms persist, see your doctor
Pain in one or both breasts, which may feel lumpy	Abnormal growth of fibrous tissue (fibroadenosis), presence of cyst or tumor	See your doctor as soon as possible
Discharge from nipple, may be yellow, greenish, blackish, or bloodstained	As above, or the release of pus from an abscess. Clear discharge normal in pregnancy	See your doctor as soon as possible
One or more lumps in breast	Fibroadenosis, cyst, or tumor	See your doctor at once
Inversion or puckering of nipple	May be normal, but it can be a symptom of cancer	See your doctor at once
Breast very small	Probably normal but may be due to failure of hormone activity in puberty, causing underdevelopment	See your doctor. In cases of hormone abnormality, treatment with hormones is possible for women aged 20 to 30
One breast bigger than the other	Small variations normal. Larger variations due to abnormal development during puberty	Hormone treatment not possible. Plastic surgery possible in severe cases. Wear padding in one bra cup

How to examine your breasts

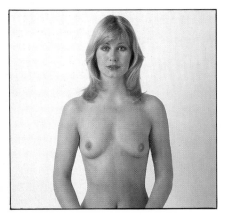

Undress to the waist and sit facing a mirror. Look for any changes in breast texture and/or size.

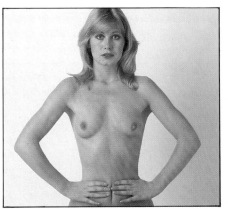

Hands on hips, shoulders back, see if nipples move up evenly, or if there is a change in breast shape.

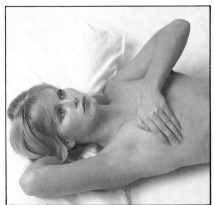

Lie down and relax. Place hands, with fingers together, gently but firmly just under the arm.

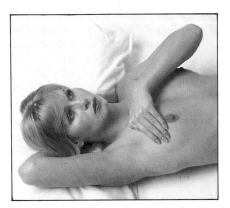

Gradually slide hand around and over breast area, moving toward the center of the chest.

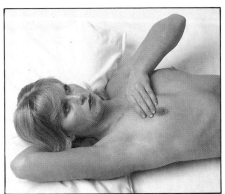

Continue this action, passing the hand completely around the breast, feeling for any sign of lumps or abnormality.

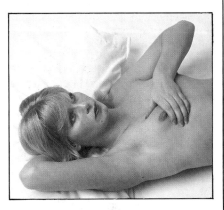

Working inward in decreasing circles, now check the nipple itself by pressing gently, again feeling for any lumps.

Brian Nash

Changes in the breasts

Just as the breasts enlarge in pregnancy, they become bigger and feel tender just before a period. This is the body's natural reaction to high levels of the hormone progesterone, present in the bloodstream at this point in the menstrual cycle. It is a healthy sign that the sexual cycle is working normally and nothing to worry about. Because it contains a synthetic progesterone, the contraceptive pill can also cause similar breast enlargement.

Other changes in the breasts are a source of great anxiety to women, because there is always a possibility that a lump discovered in the breast may turn out to be cancerous. Therefore it is always wise to report any such changes in the breasts to a doctor as soon as possible after their appearance.

The most usual sorts of lumps, however, are those due to a condition called fibroadenosis, or sclerosing adenosis, but still sometimes called by its old name,

chronic mastitis. Lumps due to this condition can occur in women from puberty onward, but they are most common toward the onset of menopause.

What happens is that the hormones cause a thickening and growth of the fibrous tissue in the breast. Often the lumps disappear after menstruation, but they should receive medical attention. Although this condition is not serious in itself, it may precede cancer.

In addition to the growth of fibrous tissue, the hormonal changes of the menstrual cycle may result in abnormal collections of fluid in the breasts. Rounded lumps, called cysts, can form. Common after the age of 40, they can cause pain, discomfort, and sometimes a bloodstained discharge from the nipple. Cysts need medical attention to distinguish them from cancer and may need to be removed surgically. Some cysts come and go with menstruation and may disappear spontaneously after a few months.

Breast tumors

Tumors of the breasts are of two kinds—benign (those that are not harmful) and malignant (those that are cancerous)—and like other breast problems, they are most likely to occur after the age of 40. All tumors are the result of cells multiplying abnormally, but while benign tumors are confined in a fibrous capsule, malignant ones are free to spread into other parts of the breast.

Typical symptoms of breast cancer include a lump in the breast that is not painful and does not change in size or consistency with the menstrual cycle, a discharge from the nipple, involution (pointing inward) of the nipple, and dimpling of the skin on the rest of the breast so that it resembles orange peel. The appearance of any one of these symptoms may have a trivial cause, but because cancer can kill, it is not worth taking even the slightest risk, so a doctor should be consulted immediately.

Breast-feeding

Q I thought that breast milk was the perfect food, but my pediatrician has suggested that I give my baby extra vitamins. Why?

A Vitamin supplements are a good idea, because both breast milk and cow's milk are somewhat deficient in vitamin D, which is necessary for proper bone development. But always consult your pediatrician about the amount you give your baby.

Q Will breast-feeding make my breasts sag afterward?

A As long as you wear a good supporting bra during pregnancy and feeding, there is no reason why your breasts should sag. Many women find that breast-feeding improves their figure.

Q When my aunt wanted to breast-feed her baby a few years ago, the nurses in the hospital were very unhelpful. In fact, she was given an injection to stop the milk before she had a chance to talk it over with them fully. Why should this happen when breast-feeding is such a good thing?

A Breast-feeding has always been subject to fashion, and your aunt may have been unlucky enough to go somewhere where those in charge held other views— or they may have simply been too short-staffed to give her the extra help she needed to get breast-feeding established. It is something that needs to be cleared up at the prenatal stage.

Q I have just had a baby and have heard stories that it is impossible to get pregnant again while breast-feeding. Is this really true?

A It is a fact that during breast-feeding your hormone balance is changed in such a way that you usually have no periods, and the release of eggs from your ovaries tends to be suppressed. But this is not a reliable method of contraception, and it is wise to take precautions against getting pregnant while breast-feeding.

Mothers who want to breast-feed should make the right preparations and know the best ways to achieve success in order to give their babies this beneficial start in life.

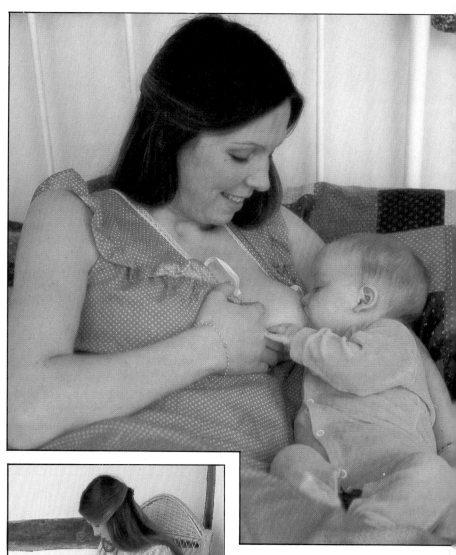

There are two basic positions for breast-feeding: either from a sitting position or lying down. But no matter which is used, the important thing is that mother and child are both comfortable.

A personal choice

While any woman who has successfully breast-fed her baby might urge other mothers to do the same, there can be no absolute rule, for there is no advantage to either the mother or the baby if the experience is not an enjoyable one or if the baby fails to take to it.

Breast-feeding undoubtedly provides the best start in life, both physically and psychologically, but these assets will quickly become tarnished if feeding the baby becomes a painful chore rather than

There is no doubt that breast-feeding has considerable advantages for a baby. But with the increasing need for women to work and the easy availability of reliable dried milk formulas, bottle-feeding has become the alternative preferred by the majority of Western women.

a chance for mutual comfort and reassurance. And even with the increasingly relaxed attitude of society toward bare breasts, even the most determined mother may find herself in potentially embarrassing situations. So the choice must be a personal one. If a woman is well prepared for the experience, aware of some of the problems that may arise, and has the support of her doctor, nurse, family, and friends, breast-feeding may be very rewarding.

Preparation

Before the baby is born, it is a good idea for the mother-to-be to see a woman actually breast-feeding—a close friend or relative, perhaps. As far as physical preparation is concerned—if the nipples are not very prominent, it may be a good idea to massage them everyday between finger and thumb in the last month of pregnancy to help them to stand out more. An application of lanolin cream every night will help to keep them supple.

If a mother wants to breast-feed, she will also need several good, supporting maternity bras that open at the front, allowing each breast to be separately exposed. Cotton is the best fabric, because it is more comfortable and absorbent than synthetic fibers. Nightclothes and shirts or dresses that fasten down the front are also more convenient and will make it easier for both mother and baby.

Size is not important

During pregnancy, the breasts become physically prepared for milk production, but no milk is actually made until after the baby is born. The milk-making potential of the breasts depends not on their actual size but on the number of glands (see Glands) they contain. So no woman needs to worry that her breasts are too small to make enough milk.

Immediately after birth the only fluid made by the breasts is colostrum, a clear liquid, rich in proteins and in antibodies, that gives the baby all it needs in the first few days and also provides invaluable protection against disease. Milk only comes into the breasts between two to five days after birth, and is mixed with colostrum at first, giving it a yellowish color. This soon turns to a pale bluish-white as the production of colostrum stops. Compared with colostrum, milk is much higher in fats and sugars and lower in proteins, but it is still a complete food.

The release, or letdown, of milk in the first week of birth, sometimes also known as the draft reflex, depends on the sucking action of the baby. Milk is secreted into the sacs, or alveoli, in the breast glands before the baby is put onto the breast. As the baby sucks, nerve messages are carried from the nipples to the hypothalamus in the brain, which in turn tells the pituitary gland to release the hormone oxytocin, which travels in the bloodstream to the alveoli. Stimulated by oxytocin, the alveoli squeeze milk into the ducts within the breast, from where it travels to reservoirs just behind the nipple, to be sucked out by the baby.

Getting started

Mothers who want to breast-feed usually want to put the baby to the breast as soon as they are able, and this may be possible immediately after the baby is delivered. If not, it should be done as soon as it can be.

A first-time mother is bound to be apprehensive, but she can relax in the knowledge that breast-feeding is a most rewarding—if demanding—experience, for which her body is perfectly adapted. The first few days before true milk comes in are valuable not just because this is the time of mutual getting to know one another. It is also when a mother finds the most comfortable position for feeding, which may be sitting or lying down.

A mother of twins can experiment to discover the best way of putting two babies to the breast at the same time. However, both babies may not always want to be fed at the same time.

Although babies will automatically suck at a nipple, they need guidance to become competent feeders. Babies are

This new mother is learning to breast-feed her baby in a relaxed, but confident, manner. On the right, she encourages the baby to grasp the nipple correctly.

born with a rooting reflex: as soon as the nipple touches the baby's cheek, he or she will instinctively turn to it and root around with the mouth until it is found. The baby should be helped by holding the nipple between the base of the index and second fingers so that he or she gets the whole nipple, with its dark surround, or areola, into its mouth. This will make sucking more efficient by helping to create a tight seal between the baby's lips and the breast and will prevent the nipple becoming sore. As the baby sucks, the mother can make sure his or her breathing is not blocked by pressing down with the index finger so that the soft breast tissue is drawn away from the nostrils.

Most mothers find that breast-feeding is difficult in the first few days after milk has come into their breasts. The initial letdown of milk may make the breasts so full that the baby cannot grasp the nipple properly, or the milk may come out so fast that the baby chokes. It may seem all too easy to give up at this early stage—especially if the baby wants to feed every two hours, or even more frequently, day and night—but these reactions are quite normal. The mother should ask for advice from those around her, and try not to feel too anxious.

Relaxation now and throughout feeding is very important, not just because breast-feeding should be a pleasure, but because anxiety can inhibit the flow of oxytocin from the brain and slow down the supply of milk. The relaxation routine that was learned before labor can be a big help at this time too. Mother and baby should settle down for each feed in peace and quiet.

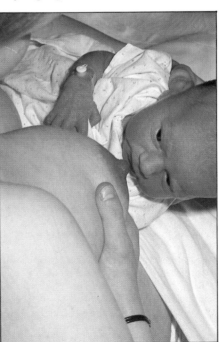

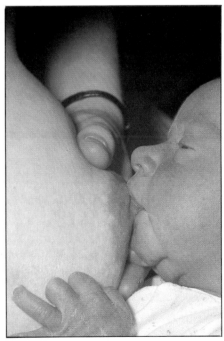

Ken Moreman

Problems and solutions

Problem	Solution/Treatment
Sore nipples	Wash and dry nipples, and apply lanolin cream after each feeding. If possible, expose nipples to the air for some time during the day. Make sure area surrounding nipple (the areola) is in the baby's mouth
Cracked nipple	Stop feeding on that side, and express the milk by hand. If problem persists more than 24 hours, see your doctor
Breast inflamed and red due to an infection	See your doctor as soon as possible, and stop feeding on that side. It should be possible to continue feeding on one side only
Lump in breast due to blocked duct	Have a hot bath, massage the breast gently toward nipple. If lump remains, see doctor as soon as possible
Nipples retracted	Pull out nipple with fingers and massage it. Wear breast shield
Breasts overfull, making it hard for baby to grasp nipple	Massage the breast toward the nipple, then squeeze the base of the nipple between finger and thumb. Try applying hot towels or ice packs to the breasts
Pains in mother's abdomen	Normal. As baby sucks, the uterus contracts. Pain will soon pass, and the contractions help uterus return to normal size
Baby reluctant to feed in first few days after birth	Stroke baby's cheek with nipple to trigger the rooting reflex. Try to feed baby before screaming is at full pitch
Baby chokes on first flow of milk into mouth	Take baby off breast until flow subsides. Place a towel under breast to mop up excess milk
Baby seems constantly hungry	Very common as milk supply is becoming established. Try to relax to increase milk flow at each feed. Make sure baby is not crying for some other reason. Consult the doctor or clinic and arrange for a test-weighing if necessary
Baby restless at breast, sucks in fits and starts	Hold the baby firmly, and try to anticipate her needs so she is not overagitated when the feeding begins. Try not to hurry
Baby falls asleep during the feeding	Try tickling toes to keep the baby awake. Lengthen intervals between feedings so that baby is more eager to feed
Baby regurgitates milk	Normal. Does not mean milk is unsuitable. Do not overfeed the baby—she may not need food every time she cries
Older brothers and sisters jealous at feeding time	Put baby and another child on your lap while feeding, and tell or read a story to older child
Father feels rejected	Involve father as much as possible in all aspects
Embarrassment	Do not get discouraged. If other people find breast-feeding offensive, go into a room where you can be alone

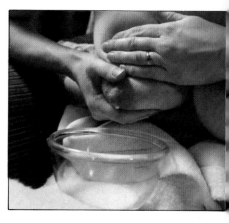

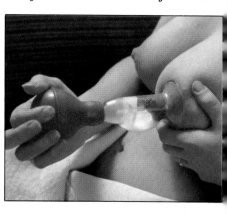

Milk may be expressed either by hand (above) or with the use of a pump (below). This is done to stimulate the supply, to allow some to be kept for a feeding when the mother is unavailable, or to clear the breast of milk when the mother cannot give milk from that breast because of soreness.

Problems with breast-feeding

One of the chief worries of nursing mothers is whether the baby is getting enough milk. Unlike bottle-fed babies, breast-fed ones regulate their own intake. The more they suck, the more milk is produced. To begin with, the baby should be allowed to suck for two minutes on each side. This time should be increased by a minute a day. The maximum length of time is determined by the baby's needs and the speed and strength of sucking.

If the nipples are sore, it may be better to give fewer, smaller feeds, because the baby gets most milk in the first minute of sucking. Remember to alternate sides so that the baby does not take the first draft from the same breast twice. Otherwise one breast will become overfull and possibly painful.

Most newborn babies need to feed every three to four hours, but unless the baby is sleepy a lot (in which case medical advice should be sought), there is no need to wake a sleeping baby for a feed.

In the early days of breast-feeding, a woman can help to stimulate her milk supply by expressing the remaining milk from the breast after feeding with a special pump or by squeezing milk out by hand, starting from the edge of the breast and working toward the nipple. The milk can be collected in a bowl and stored in the refrigerator, and if not needed by the

baby, it will be received gladly by any hospital with a premature baby unit. Later on, expressing milk can be very useful if a mother wants to leave her baby for several hours but does not want him or her to have any other kind of milk. Good care should be taken of the breasts by keeping the nipples clean and dry and applying lanolin cream twice a day to keep them supple.

Outlook

All mothers find caring for a new baby exhausting, but there is no reason why breast-feeding should be any more tiring than bottle-feeding as long as the mother is generally fit and eats a good diet.

If all goes well, breast-feeding can continue until the baby is ready to drink from a cup with a spout, usually after the age of six months. As he or she gets used to this, successive feeds can be dropped. But a mother should never feel a failure if she gives her baby an occasional bottle or if circumstances prevent her from breast-feeding; nor should she worry that her baby will be psychologically damaged if she does not breast-feed.

Breath-holding

Q Are little girls more liable to have breath-holding attacks than little boys?

A No. They can occur in either sex, but are generally more likely to happen with boys.

Q I'm convinced that my small son holds his breath just to frighten me. Is this, in fact, dangerous?

A You may be right if he is very strong willed—but there is no risk of him doing himself lasting harm, and the condition should cure itself as he gets older.

Q My neighbor's children have never had breath-holding attacks, so she says. But when she saw my child do this, she said it was the way I brought him up. Could this be so?

A Your neighbor was just lucky. About one child in eight does this, but they usually grow out of it by the age of four. However, you may want to spend more time with your child, as he may be trying to call attention to himself.

Q If I don't give my small daughter exactly what she wants, she starts holding her breath. How can I make her stop?

A The best thing to do is to keep calm and try to ignore the growing storm. If you are in a public place, like a supermarket, it is best to pick her up, pay the bill, and leave as rapidly as possible. Under no circumstances give her what she wants to keep her quiet— this will only encourage her to repeat the performance.

Q Although I don't usually approve of using physical punishment, my mother tells me I should slap my son's face when he starts acting up and holding his breath. Is this really a good idea?

A Slapping may relieve your own feelings of frustration, but there is nothing particularly beneficial in this action, and it is unlikely to be effective in preventing your son's breath-holding tactics.

Young children sometimes turn blue in the face when they are angry—but this is not as alarming as it may seem.

When toddlers are beside themselves with anger, frustration, or fear—perhaps over something that seems very trivial— they very often react by holding their breath. An attack can occur in children between the ages of one and three years, and they seem to affect boys more than girls. It can be the culmination of a temper tantrum, be triggered by pain, or by an overwhelming need for attention.

When it starts, the child cries out loudly two or three times, breathes out and stops. His face turns blue. In the mildest cases this lasts for five to ten seconds, after which the child quickly recovers as though nothing had happened. Sometimes the breath-holding continues for up to 20 seconds, the child's face becomes leaden, then turns pale; he loses consciousness and goes limp, crumpling to the ground. Being unconscious, he automatically takes a breath, recovers consciousness, and after one faint cry, continues at full volume. In a few moments he is back to normal.

Even less common, breathing is suspended for half a minute or more: when this happens, the child turns rigid after the limp stage and then has a convulsion, rather like an epileptic seizure; but although this is frightening to watch, it is actually not very serious. The child soon recovers his breathing and his senses, although he may be confused or drowsy for a little while after the attack, which he will probably not remember.

Strong emotions

An adult who is upset may become speechless with anger. An emotion that we are unable to express makes us decide to hold back from saying anything. When a child feels a strong emotion that he cannot express, it sets off the same reaction but goes beyond his control.

Holding his breath for more than five seconds depletes his blood of oxygen: it becomes blue and so does his face. However, the buildup of carbon dioxide, the waste gas produced as the tissues use up oxygen, automatically stimulates the respiratory center: a built-in safety arrangement. Obviously, if a child is anemic and his blood has less oxygen-carrying capacity, even a few seconds' breath-holding will result in a noticeable attack. If your child does have a severe attack, take him to your doctor to be checked for anemia.

What brings on breath-holding

Many emotions can start a breath-holding attack in a toddler. For instance, he may be angry if another child grabs his toy or tries to do so; he may feel frustrated— maybe he is in his playpen and something has caught his eye outside that he cannot reach; he may feel thwarted because an adult refuses to let him have or do what he wants; or he may simply be frightened of something.

Breath-holding is one of the ways in which a toddler may express strong emotions.

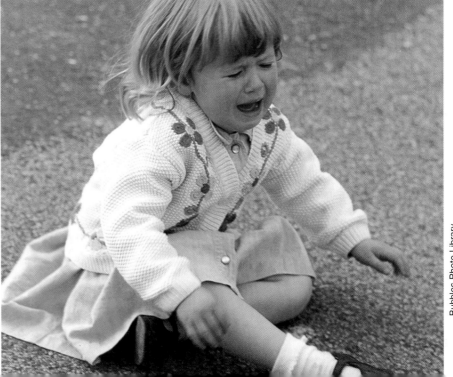

Breathing

Breathing is an essential, life-supporting activity. This makes it vital to preserve the health of the nose, throat, bronchial tubes, and lungs—and to insure that any problems receive early treatment.

Q Does smoking really cause lung cancer? My husband smokes 40 cigarettes a day. Should I get him to cut down?

A Although lung cancer does not only affect smokers, and not all smokers contract it, there is a relationship. Lung cancer is the most common form of cancer among smokers, and the more a person smokes, the higher the risk will be.

All cancers are normal body cells that are no longer under control. They do nothing but reproduce and begin to act like a parasite. The continual intake of tobacco smoke causes cells to behave in this way. Eventually the cancer cells outnumber the neighboring cells and form a tumor in the bronchial tubes—the bronchi—or deeper in the lungs. To convince your husband, point out the number of doctors who have stopped.

If he is motivated to stop, he may be helped with the physical part by taking nicotine in the form of chewing gum or using a skin patch. This treatment should continue for a few weeks after quitting.

Q I have a tendency to get bronchitis. If I leave the windows in the bedroom open at night, will this help?

A Bronchitis often begins as an infection in the nose and throat, followed by a chest infection. The bronchi are more prone to infection if they are irritated by tobacco smoke, noxious fumes, and cold air. If there are smokers in the house, opening a window may remove some of the smoke. However, cold air and pollution coming in through the window, especially in cities, are just as bad. It is better to leave windows closed at night: warm atmospheres are best for all bronchial conditions.

Q My son has been diagnosed as having small lungs. Is this a serious condition?

A Each lung has a capacity of about 0.09 cubic feet (2.5 liters), but the amount of air passing in and out of the lungs is often only a tenth of this. Your son should be all right. Indeed many people manage well with one lung.

Awake or asleep, humans breathe an average of 12 times a minute and in 24 hours breathe in and breathe out more than 282 cu ft (8,000 liters) of air. During heavy physical exercise, the breathing rate will increase to up to 80 times a minute.

Why breathing is necessary

The purpose of moving so much air in and out of the body is to enable the lungs to do two things: to extract the oxygen needed to sustain life and to rid the body of carbon dioxide, the waste product of internal chemical processes.

Before the air reaches the lungs, however, it passes through a series of filters to purify it. The fresh air of the countryside contains bacteria, fungal spores, and dust, and the town or city dweller has additional pollution to contend with. But although the body is equipped with a series of traps and filters to deal with both situations, it is not a totally fail-safe system, and illnesses can and do result, particularly if people smoke or work in industries where they are exposed to certain kinds of dust.

Early development

The respiratory system begins to develop early on in the growth of the fetus, the branching pattern of the airways and arteries being complete by the sixteenth week after conception. At 28 weeks, cells that secrete surfactant, a fluid, start to develop in the lungs, preventing them from sticking together. The vital gas-exchanging parts of the lungs, where oxygen is absorbed into the bloodstream and carbon waste dioxide removed, then remain filled with fluid until the baby is born.

This fluid can be a problem in premature babies, who are often not strong enough to breathe deeply, which would inflate the lungs, allowing the fluid to disperse. In full-term babies, most parts of the respiratory system are fully developed. However, it is not until the age of eight that the gas-exchanging part of the lung in children, whether premature or full-term, is fully formed.

Inhaling

Inhaled and exhaled air goes through the nose and mouth. As air enters the nose, dust particles and other foreign bodies are trapped by coarse hairs. The air continues its passage into the nasal cavity, where the moist membrane that lines the walls warms the air and produces mucus to collect even more particles of dirt. Hairlike projections on the membrane called cilia, are continually in motion pushing the film of mucus and its trapped contents back toward the throat to be swallowed.

At the back of the nasal cavity and above the mouth lie two sets of lymph glands: the tonsils (see Tonsils) and the adenoids. Because their role is to pick up and destroy invading bacteria, they often become infected and swollen, causing tonsillitis. A sustained buildup of invading bacteria also creates the swelling and irritation of the throat that is a symptom of colds and bouts of flu.

From the throat, the filtered, moistened, and warmed air passes into the windpipe (the trachea), where, as in the nasal cavity, cilia waft the mucous layer and its contents toward the throat for disposal by swallowing. Once past the trachea, the inhaled air has received all the screening it will receive before passing into the lungs, where oxygen from it is absorbed into the bloodstream.

At its lower end, the windpipe divides into two smaller tubes called the bronchi, one leading to each lung. It is here that infections, such as those that cause bronchitis and pneumonia, can build up and cause breathing problems.

In the lungs

Within the lungs each bronchus divides into smaller tubes, the bronchioles; these in turn branch and form millions of tiny air sacs, the alveoli—each surrounded by

Right: Air inhaled via the trachea, bronchi, and bronchioles reaches the alveoli, where oxygen from the air is transferred to the capillaries surrounding each alveolus. The oxygenated blood is carried to the pulmonary vein and into the left side of the heart and pushed into the aorta. Blood then moves around the body, through arteries to the capillaries. The oxygen carried by the red blood cells is given to the tissue cells, which transfer their waste product, carbon dioxide, to the red cells. This is carried back through the veins into the right side of the heart, and finally, the blood flows out through the pulmonary artery and into the lungs. At the site of the alveoli, the circulating blood gives up its carbon dioxide, which is exhaled, and takes in oxygen again

How oxygen is carried around the body and carbon dioxide is removed

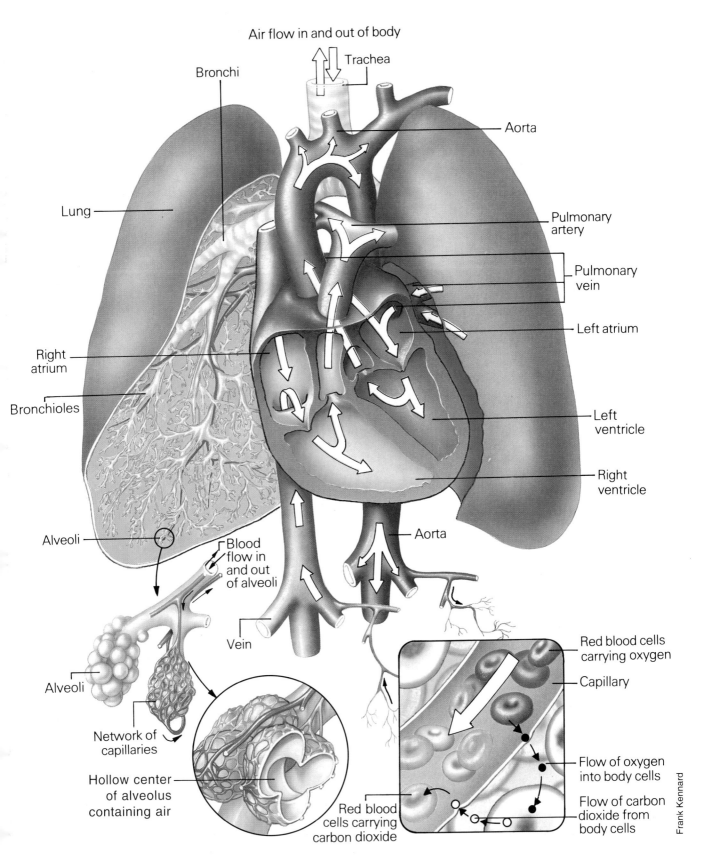

Air flow in and out of body

Trachea

Bronchi

Aorta

Lung

Pulmonary artery

Pulmonary vein

Left atrium

Right atrium

Bronchioles

Left ventricle

Right ventricle

Alveoli

Blood flow in and out of alveoli

Aorta

Vein

Alveoli

Network of capillaries

Hollow center of alveolus containing air

Red blood cells carrying carbon dioxide

Red blood cells carrying oxygen

Capillary

Flow of oxygen into body cells

Flow of carbon dioxide from body cells

Frank Kennard

a meshwork of fine capillaries (see Capillaries)—where the exchange of oxygen and carbon dioxide takes place. The branches of the pulmonary artery carry carbon dioxide-rich blood, and this gas is given up in return for the oxygen in the new air that has entered the alveolar sacs. The lungs then exhale the carbon dioxide in the deoxygenated air along with a certain amount of water vapor that comes from the moist membranes of the alveoli. On cold days this water vapor condenses and shows up as steaming breath.

The lungs fill most of the chest cavity and are inflated and deflated by muscular movements of the chest and the rise and fall of a sheet of muscle, the diaphragm, that lies under the ribs and divides the chest cavity from the abdomen.

Each lung is surrounded by a double membrane, the pleura. The outer pleura is attached to the chest walls and the diaphragm; the inner pleura attaches itself to each lung. Between the two membranes is a cavity; a thin film of fluid on its surface protects the delicate tissues as they move against each other as the lungs inflate and deflate. Inflammation of the pleura, a condition called pleurisy, causes pain when inhaling or coughing.

Exhaling

When breathing normally, the diaphragm (see Diaphragm) does most of the work. The muscle contracts, and the volume of the chest cavity increases. The ribs are pulled upward and outward by muscles, called intercostals, that lie between them, and as the pressure within the lungs drops, air is sucked in. Breathing out is a passive process: the diaphragm and the intercostal muscles relax, and the natural elasticity of the lung tissue forces air out.

Breathing rates

Breathing is controlled by the respiratory center of the brain, the medulla oblongata, and is regulated according to the levels of carbon dioxide in the blood rather than the amount of oxygen present. The brain will respond to an increased production of carbon dioxide, such as during a period of physical exercise, and adjust the breathing rate accordingly. Breathing will become deeper and faster so that, as more oxygen is inhaled, stimulating the heartbeat, blood flow will increase and the carbon dioxide will be burned off. Once the exercise ceases, the carbon dioxide level falls and breathing will return to normal.

Voluntary alterations in breathing rates occur during activities such as talking, singing, and eating. Yawning, sighing, coughing, and hiccuping involve still other kinds of respiration. Laughing and crying, both of which involve long breaths followed by short bursts of exhalation, are respiratory changes due to emotional stimuli.

Holding your breath, either deliberately (when swimming underwater) or unwittingly (as a result of an attack of nerves), also alters the breathing pattern. The carbon dioxide level falls after the first few deep breaths, which are then held, and the brain ceases to be stimulated. This can lead to a blackout, and when swimming underwater, death by drowning if the person cannot return to the surface. On the other hand, high altitude sickness may occur when the unacclimatized person climbs to high altitudes. The body tissues may become unoxygenated, and the person feels giddy, nauseous, and as he or she goes higher, there will be a feeling of sublime indifference, called euphoria; loss of muscular coordination;

and eventually, unconsciousness, if the person does not either receive oxygen or make a rapid descent at the onset of these symptoms.

Mechanisms of injury

Although subject to many different forms of injury, the lungs have only a few basic ways of reacting. Assaults as varied as inhaled toxic gases, drugs, viruses, or lack of oxygen due to shock, trauma, or mountain sickness all produce a profound outpouring of fluid into the alveoli (pulmonary edema), which may effectively drown the patient if untreated. Bacterial infections cause the alveoli to fill with pus, while chronic bronchitis cause

These magnified cilia, which line the inside of the nasal passages, are trapping tiny particles of dust.

Breathing disorders

Symptoms	Condition	Action
Runny eyes and nose, coughing, sneezing, sore throat, and headache	Common cold	Colds rarely last for more than a week but, if they persist, can lead to complications such as bronchitis. There is no known cure, but aspirin or antihistamine may make the symptoms less uncomfortable. Keep warm and stay indoors. Antibiotics will not help, but drinking fluids may
Chills, high fever, pain in tonsil area, difficulty swallowing, headache, pain in jaw and neck. Tonsils red, enlarged, spotted	Tonsillitis	Antibiotic or sulfonamide drugs; cold drinks or food (ice cream). Seek medical attention; if severe or untreated, can lead to other diseases, such as rheumatic fever
Dry, irritating cough with thick, yellow mucus and light fever. Cough persists for up to two weeks	Acute bronchitis	Rest in bed in a humid room with inhalants, plenty of hot drinks. Stimulant cough medicine by day and a sedative one at night
Constant, vigorous cough that is worse in the mornings than in the evenings. Clear sputum that may become yellow if a secondary infection sets in	Chronic bronchitis	Antibiotics to prevent secondary infection, breathing exercises, clean air, and no smoking. Immediate treatment of any other respiratory ailments
Shortness of breath, difficulty in breathing, tight chest, wheezing, sweating	Asthma	Test for allergies or infection. Treat with appropriate drugs. Breathing exercises and bronchodilators also give relief. Avoid stressful situations and catching colds or other respiratory infections. Prolonged attacks require hospitalization
Pain caused by coughing, breathing heavily, or moving. The pain may occur in the shoulder if the pleura covering the diaphragm is affected	Pleurisy	Almost always caused by a virus or bacterial infection; often associated with pneumonia. Appropriate treatment for the infection should be prescribed, along with painkillers

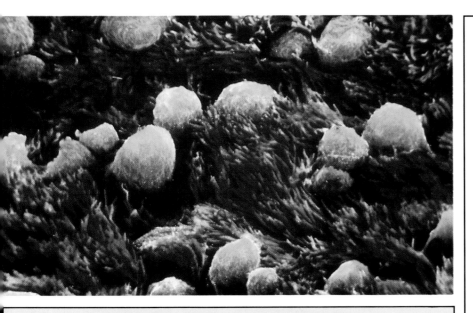

Breathing disorders

Symptoms	Condition	Action
Sudden fever, chest pains, cough and bloodstained sputum, sweating, shivering, and often vomiting and diarrhea	Pneumonia	Rest in bed, antibiotics, and breathing exercises under your doctor's direction
Children: Fever, swollen lymph glands in the chest, weight loss, coughing, and breathlessness *Adults:* Fever, heavy sweating at night, fatigue, weight loss, coughing up blood-tinged sputum, and possible pleurisy	Tuberculosis	Drugs clear up most infections quite quickly. More serious forms require hospital treatment for up to three months and prescribed drugs for up to 18 months after
Increasing feeling of constriction of the chest and breathlessness. Frequent coughing attacks and production of sputum	Emphysema	Emphysema is the consequence of respiratory ailments like chronic bronchitis and pneumoconiosis. Treatment consists of clean air, no smoking, and breathing exercises. Severe cases may need oxygen before physical activity or sleep
Spitting blood, coughing, and breathlessness. Possibly asthma	Pneumoconiosis	Pneumoconiosis means any lung disease caused by inhaling dust particles. Some dusts are harmless, but silica and asbestos cause damage to the lung tissue and early treatment is essential
Coughing with sputum that may be bloodstained. Later pneumonia and partial lung collapse, followed by weakness, weight loss, and lethargy	Lung cancer	Surgical removal of the tumor is possible, and radiotherapy and drug therapy are the usual treatments
Sudden onset of high fever, followed by croupy, nonproductive cough, then thick phlegm in the bronchi and trachea. Extreme shortness of breath	Laryngotracheobronchitis (croup)	If in a child, urgent medical attention advised. Antibiotics given, sometimes hospitalization necessary. Keep room warm, take prescribed drugs

progressive destruction of the bronchial walls. However, all these conditions, if not stopped soon enough or cured, progress in a similar fashion to the destruction of functioning lung tissue and its replacement with fibrous scars. This severely impairs the individual's ability to transfer oxygen to the blood.

Prevention of disorders is therefore important. An individual should be aware of toxic materials in the workplace or living environment and take suitable precautions. A cough that brings up mucus and does not clear up in a week or two, should be treated by a doctor. Above all it is best not to take up smoking, and existing smokers should make every effort to stop, since cigarette smoke alone (or acting with any of the above agents) is probably the single most destructive factor in causing chronic lung disease.

There are many treatments and therapies available that can help curb a smoking habit. Chewing gum (with added nicotine) and skin patches (through which the nicotine is absorbed into the skin) can help to wean the body off cigarettes. Hypnosis, acupuncture, and meditation can also be effective.

Breech birth

Q One week I am told that my baby is breech and the next that it is lying head down. The last ultrasound scan showed it in breech; does this mean it will be born upside down?

A Not necessarily. Even the most experienced obstetrician or nurse-midwife can make a mistake, and the baby can change its position several times before engaging either the right or the wrong way around. Until you are told the baby is definitely breech in the last few weeks, it is best to forget about its position altogether.

Q My doctor wants to turn my baby around because it is breech. But I'm not sure I want her to do it. What are the dangers involved?

A Ask your doctor why she wants to turn the baby; there may be a special reason relevant to your medical history. On the whole, because breech births are now so much safer, many obstetricians prefer not to take the risk of turning a breech baby around. In rare cases the water can break, inducing a premature birth; the umbilical cord can also be pulled accidentally, and any decrease in the supply of oxygen could have serious consequences.

Q My last baby was born breech. Does this mean that my next baby will be born in the same manner?

A It is possible that this might be the case with a subsequent birth, but it would have nothing to do with your first child having been a breech and would be a pure coincidence.

Q When a baby's bottom is born first, doesn't the shock cause the baby to inhale mucus during birth?

A The cord joining the mother and baby remains a life-support system until the baby actually leaves the mother's body and is able to breathe in air. It is normal for a baby to inhale mucus anyway as the head is born, and this rarely requires any medical treatment.

Babies are usually born headfirst. When one arrives feet, knees, or bottom first, this is known as a breech birth. Today there need be no cause for alarm, because the risk of complications is minimal.

Approximately 3 to 4 percent of babies enter the world bottom first; knee and foot presentations are rarer still. As a result of modern screening tests during pregnancy, women today usually know in advance whether a breech birth is expected, so any risks can be minimized. Many of these babies are delivered by Caesarean section (an operation where the baby is lifted out through an incision made in the mother's abdomen), but a normal vaginal delivery is possible.

Causes

There are certain circumstances in which a breech birth is more likely to occur. For example, when a multiple birth is expected, it is more than likely that at least one of the babies will be breech; twins often present themselves as one headfirst (cephalic) and the other breech.

A breech birth can also be the result of an abnormality in the pregnancy, but this is usually picked up early and plans for the birth made accordingly. Such a problem is the retention of excessive fluid around the baby, a condition called hydramnios. This fluid—called liquor—permits ease of movement, but the more there is around the baby, the greater the likelihood of the baby being in the breech position at birth.

Many women produce an excessive amount of liquor for no reason and go on to produce perfectly healthy babies, despite the fact that they are statistically more likely to have a breech birth than women who do not have hydramnios.

It is normal for a woman to notice changes in her baby's position from mid-pregnancy onward. At midpregnancy, there is more fluid in relation to the size of the baby, but as the baby grows, there is progressively less room for movement (except in cases of hydramnios).

Since there is still a fair amount of room for the baby to move around at seven months, many premature babies are born breech. But at about eight months (36 weeks), the presenting part of the fetus normally sinks into the pelvis, a position called engagement; once this occurs there is no further movement. At this stage, doctors can predict the birth position of the baby.

Symptoms

Many women who have a breech birth are able to feel their baby's head pressing

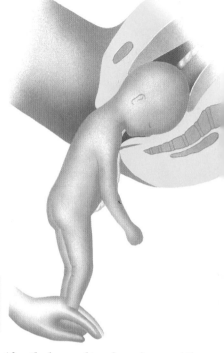

Venner Artists

After the legs and trunk are born and the shoulders have been rotated out, the baby's body is allowed to hang down, causing flexion (bending) of the head.

under their lower ribs toward the end of their pregnancy. This can be very uncomfortable, particularly when sitting down. Once the bottom slips into the pelvis, however, this discomfort will ease. Unfortunately engagement does not always occur at 36 weeks, especially if the mother has already had a child, and this pressure can persist right up to the time of the actual birth.

On the whole a pregnancy that results in a breech birth will progress like any other. But it will differ in one or two ways, and in the last month, when the bottom engages into the pelvis, the doctor will take special precautions to insure the safe delivery of the baby. He or she will check the dates to make sure the baby does not have extra time for growth beyond the calculated delivery date; this avoids the head being too big to pass easily through the pelvis.

Special tests

Most pregnant women these days are examined under an ultrasound scanner as part of their normal prenatal care. This machine measures the size of the baby

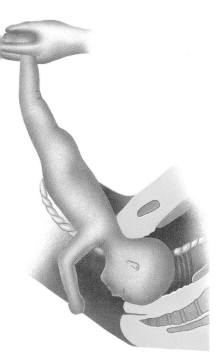

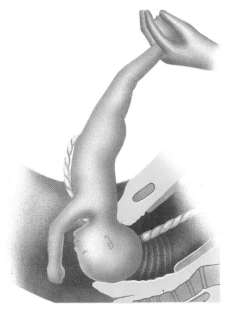

The rest of the baby's head emerges and is now born slowly.

Once the hairline and nape of the neck emerge, the body is raised so that the face appears.

and can prove particularly useful in estimating the size of a breech baby's head in order to insure a safe and easy journey through the pelvis. For this reason the pelvis is usually measured too.

Both checks can be done by X ray, but this technique is no longer advised: there is a small risk of the fetus becoming contaminated by minute amounts of radiation. If scanning tests are not conclusive, however, or there is no alternative, an X ray may be carried out as a last resort.

The first stage of labor

Labor can be longer when a baby is breech, due mainly to the presenting part of the body not acting as efficiently on the neck of the womb (the cervix) as a hard head does. The cervix will open well in response to the descending head, but if it is a softer part, such as the bottom, labor can take much longer. If a knee or elbow presents itself first, then labor will be held up considerably; if there is no progress at all—as can easily happen in either of the last two cases—a Caesarean section may have to be performed.

If a woman knows she is going to have a breech birth, it is wise for her to discuss the types of pain relief available with the doctor or nurse-midwife before going into labor. Many obstetricians (doctors specializing in pregnancy and birth) advise having an epidural—an anesthetic that is injected into the epidural space

just in front of the spinal cord. This has the effect of numbing the whole area and will help a woman through a long, exhausting labor. An epidural will also relieve any discomfort felt in the birth canal when the baby's head is being delivered with lift-out forceps. This is an instrument used in most breech deliveries today as a safety measure to protect the head from possible damage.

In a normal labor, with a cephalic, or headfirst, presentation, the mother-to-be is not allowed any fluids by mouth; in a breech birth, this policy is even more rigidly enforced in case the need to give a general anesthetic arises.

If the labor is likely to be long, an intravenous drip of dextrose—a mixture of water and glucose—is given in the early stages of the delivery. This will prevent the woman's blood being depleted of sugar, which would make her tire early.

If an epidural has been chosen as a method to relieve pain, a drip may be necessary to counteract any side effects that may occur. Some women, for example, will suffer a drop in their blood pressure as a direct result of having had an epidural, but this situation can be improved by using a dextrose drip.

The second stage of labor

A great amount of skill is required in safely dealing with a breech birth. The correct time of the birth must be gauged; then the baby is carefully guided into the world, with the obstetrician usually delivering the baby's head with forceps to prevent accidental injury.

When the cervix is finally fully dilated, the doctor will be able to see the presenting part of the baby's body: the bottom, an arm, or a leg. To allow easy passage for the baby, and so that the delivery of the head can be controlled and the head lifted clear with forceps, a small cut, called an episiotomy, is made in the perineum, the area between the vaginal entrance and the anus.

As the buttocks descend, the legs will ease out gently. If they are extended, the knees can be gently eased and flexed by the doctor. The cord is checked to insure it is not compressed at this stage and then watched carefully throughout the rest of the labor.

The weight of the baby's body will draw down the shoulders, which will naturally rotate. With luck, it may well not be necessary to touch the baby. Then, as the woman pushes, the shoulders and head should follow, and the baby can then be lifted up to allow the airways to clear.

If a breech birth goes well, the body of the baby will emerge in its own time— slowly and safely. The one danger is at the end, when there is a danger of the head being born too fast. The woman may give an unexpected push, causing the head to suffer a sudden pressure, and hence possible damage and internal bleeding. The medical staff will therefore watch carefully, and if there is any danger of the head following the body too fast, forceps will be used to hold back the head and bring it into the world more gently.

If all goes well, the umbilical cord, which is still attached to the mother and child, will be cut, the placenta and membranes delivered, and finally, the episiotomy stitched up.

The baby is then checked thoroughly by the pediatrician, who is always on hand during a breech birth. As there is always the slight risk of internal bleeding in the baby if its head is delivered too fast, it may be given an injection of vitamin K to help the blood to clot.

Outlook

In most cases of breech birth the baby is usually handed to the mother once it has been checked. If there are complications —and these days, this is a rare occurrence—then the baby may need to be observed for a short while in an intensive-care nursery. Most of these allow the parents to spend the maximum amount of time with their baby, and the mother is allowed to breast-feed.

Most hospitals will allow the father to stay for the birth. He can ask questions as the delivery progresses, and this way both partners can be sure of understanding just what is happening at every stage of the baby's arrival.

Bronchitis

Bronchitis, which can become chronic, is a serious infection of the lungs and bronchial tubes. Breathing polluted air and smoking are mainly responsible.

Q I sometimes feel a little better after coughing in the morning. Since I am a heavy smoker, does that mean that I am in the early stages of bronchitis?

A What you describe does not necessarily mean you have bronchitis, although smoking does contribute enormously to the disease. Heavy smokers may believe that a cigarette in the morning will "cut the phlegm," but this is nonsense.

Q My uncle has difficulty in walking very far—even to the other end of the backyard. He blames this on his bronchitis. Is he right?

A Yes. Generally speaking the worse the bronchitis, the less exercise the person can tolerate. Doctors tend to divide bronchitis into four stages: 1, a slight cough in the morning but no other trouble; 2, breathless on exertion; 3, so breathless that the patient is unable to leave the house; and 4, so breathless that the patient is unable to conduct a normal conversation.

Q Does bronchitis cause cancer?

A No. But the smoking that causes chronic bronchitis is a potent cause of cancer. If you smoke more than 20 cigarettes a day, you increase your chances of developing lung cancer 20 times and your chances of getting chronic bronchitis 50 times.

Q If I give up smoking tomorrow, will my chronic bronchitis get better?

A It is possible that the course of the disease may be slowed, and in some cases actually arrested by giving up smoking, but the bronchitis is never reversed. Of course your overall health will be improved by kicking the habit, so it is definitely worth trying to stop. Ask your family doctor for help and guidance. Nicotine gum and patches, available from the drugstore, have helped some people to quit.

Bronchitis is an inflammation of the main bronchial tubes—the bronchi—caused by a bacterial or viral infection. It may develop suddenly, following a head cold (acute bronchitis), or it may persist or return regularly for many years, causing progressive degeneration of the bronchi and lungs (chronic bronchitis).

Those at risk

Certain people are more susceptible than others: men are more so than women, outnumbering them 10 to one. The reasons why are unclear. Smokers are 50 times more likely to get chronic bronchitis than nonsmokers.

Recent estimates suggest that 14.6 million Americans suffer from chronic bronchitis or bronchitis and its common sequel, emphysema. These diseases cause 80,000 deaths every year and rank fifth as the cause of death in the US. Eighty to 90 percent of cases are caused by cigarette smoking. The risk of death from these causes is 30 times greater for people who smoke more than 25 cigarettes per day than for nonsmokers.

A person with severe obstructive lung disease suffers from constant breathlessness, even at rest, is unable to undertake any exertion, and often has to use the neck and shoulder muscles in an exhausting attempt to get enough breath. Despite this, and although it may deprive them of up to 8 percent of the oxygen-carrying capacity of the blood, a sizable propor-

tion of these people still continue to smoke cigarettes.

In people who smoke, the probability of developing chronic bronchitis increases with age, and thus with the number of cigarettes smoked. More than half of all middle-aged men who smoke a pack of cigarettes a day or more have a persistent cough with sputum. People who quit continue to have a greater liability to chronic bronchitis than nonsmokers, but this is less than that of current smokers. This liability declines gradually with time. Cigar and pipe smokers also are likely to develop chronic bronchitis, but the risk is significantly lower than that of smokers.

Causes

Generally bronchitis occurs with greater frequency in winter, in damp, cold climates, and in heavily polluted environments. Chilling, overcrowding, and fatigue are contributory factors.

Most cases of acute bronchitis arise from a viral infection that spreads to the chest. Chronic bronchitis causes irritation and coughing. The lungs lose their elasticity, and the exchange of vital oxygen, which is breathed in, and carbon dioxide waste, which is breathed out, is impaired. The bronchial tubes become permanently inflamed, and this results in an increased production of mucus from specialized cells in the walls of the bronchi, called goblet cells. The mucus coughed up is called sputum (phlegm).

How bronchitic mucus affects the respiratory system

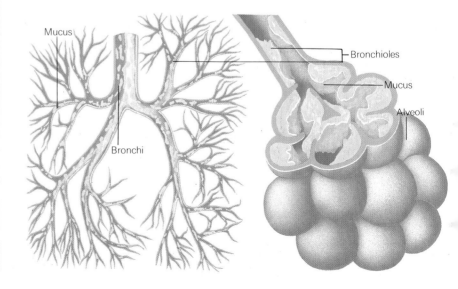

Mucus

Bronchi

Bronchioles

Mucus

Alveoli

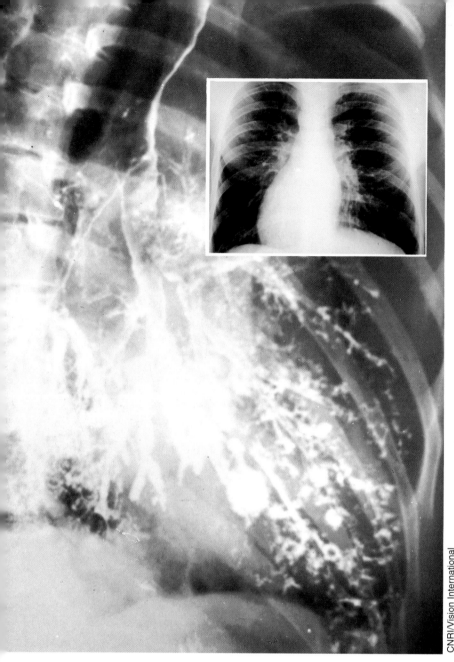

The alveoli in this lung of a person with chronic bronchitis are grossly swollen. A normal, clear lung is inset (right).

Because it is difficult to look at the bronchi directly, doctors rely on the chief symptom, sputum production, in order to make a diagnosis. The color of the sputum shows how serious the form of chronic bronchitis is.

Symptoms

In acute bronchitis the initial symptoms are a head cold, runny nose, fever and chills, aching muscles, and possibly back pain. This is soon followed by the most obvious feature: a persistent cough. At first it is dry and racking, but it becomes phlegmy. It is worse at night and when the person breathes in smoke and fumes.

The main characteristic of chronic bronchitis is, again, a cough with sputum, often occurring in paroxysms. Other symptoms depend on how much, or how little, emphysema is present. This disorder causes the lungs to become overstretched, making breathing out difficult.

A person with chronic bronchitis and no emphysema tends to be overweight and have a bluish tinge to his or her lips due to cyanosis (a bluish color in the blood caused by lack of oxygen). Shortness of breath occurs only during exercise. A person with bronchitis and a great deal of emphysema, who has lost a lot of his or her oxygen-exchanging ability, is short of breath at all times. People with bronchitis and emphysema tend to be underweight and, as the disease worsens, develop a barrel chest. The person with chronic bronchitis also wheezes.

Studies of autopsy findings of large numbers of people have shown that some discernible degree of emphysematous change is present in the lungs of 65 percent of men and 15 percent of women. A degree sufficient to lead to symptoms and a clinical diagnosis of emphysema, however, is present in less than one percent of the population. Clinical emphysema does not occur in nonsmokers, is present in 12 percent of people who smoke less than one pack a day, long term, and is also present in nearly 20 percent of those who smoke one or more packs a day.

Treatment

The best treatment for acute bronchitis is bed rest in a warm room. Aspirin will reduce the fever, and cough medicines will relieve the cough. Antibiotics may be needed if the cause is bacterial.

Treatment of chronic bronchitis is more difficult. The patient's lungs are already damaged, and the obstruction of the airways is not easily reversible.

CNRI/Vision International

Types of bronchitis

Causes	Symptoms	Action
Acute bronchitis		
• Bacteria or virus infection, often following a cold • Smoking	Head cold; runny nose; fever and chills; aching muscles Persistent cough: initially dry and racking; later loose and producing sputum	Bed rest; warm atmosphere; aspirin; cough medicine; fluids; antibiotics Stop smoking
Chronic bronchitis		
• Persistent irritation of the bronchial tubes; bacterial infection; irritation to damaged bronchial tubes and lungs. • Smoking; wet, cold climates; pollution; low resistance; and fatigue	Sputum, cough; wheezing Bronchitis with emphysema: shortness of breath; weight loss; barrel chest Bronchitis without emphysema: shortness of breath when exercising; weight gain; bluish tinge to lips	Stop smoking. Bronchial dilator drugs; physiotherapy of chest; postural drainage; yoga and breathing exercises; antibiotics. Severe cases may require hospitalization; oxygen, if necessary. Avoid bronchial irritants

Q I have never smoked but have been recently diagnosed as having chronic bronchitis. Will this lead to emphysema?

A No, it is not likely. Although chronic bronchitis can be caused and made worse by smoking, it can be due to other factors such as air pollution and industrial irritants. But clinical emphysema does not develop in those who have never smoked. It only occurs in smokers, and the likelihood increases with the amount of cigarettes smoked. Its long-term effects are present in 12 percent of those who smoke up to one pack a day, and in those who smoke between one and two packs a day, its occurrence is up to around 20 percent.

Q My uncle is constantly puffing on a pipe. Is it usual for pipe smokers to develop bronchitis?

A Those who smoke cigars and pipes are much less likely to develop chronic bronchitis than those who smoke cigarettes, but if your uncle is worried, he should try and cut down on his pipe smoking. There is still some chance that he may suffer from the disease, as well as mouth and lung cancers.

Q Is bronchitis a disease that can result in death?

A Most definitely. In the United States, bronchitis ranks number five as the most common cause of death, resulting in around 80,000 fatalities per year. Between 80 and 90 percent of all cases of the disease are caused by smoking. It cannot be stated often enough—if you don't smoke, don't start; if you do smoke, quit.

Q My sister has bronchitis. Can she borrow my asthma inhaler in an emergency?

A Many people with bronchitis are prescribed a bronchial dilator, the same type of medicine that is used for asthma. But it is best if your sister sees a doctor so that she gets the proper treatment for her particular condition and her own inhaler.

Bronchial dilator drugs may be given to relieve any such obstruction, while physiotherapy will help the patient get rid of any sputum. Postural drainage can also be tried: the patient lies on a bed, a large cushion raising the groin and smaller pillows supporting the chest. Tapping the chest in this position causes the patient to cough up sputum. Yoga (see Yoga) and breathing exercises generally may ease shortness of breath. In severe cases urgent hospital treatment may be required. Oxygen might have to be given through the course of the illness.

The best form of relief is to remove as many bronchial irritants as possible. The patient should stop smoking immediately; although chronic bronchitis cannot be reversed, it can be arrested. Those with chronic bronchitis should try to avoid environments where there are irritants, because these can bring on attacks.

Outlook

With acute bronchitis, the fever may last as long as five days and the coughing for weeks after; but if the patient receives treatment and takes sensible precautions, the illness will simply run its course and the outlook is good.

Chronic bronchitis is more serious. It is a degenerative disease, particularly when combined with emphysema, and can result in death due to respiratory failure, when there is insufficient oxygen in the blood. One of the most important complications is carbon dioxide narcosis (stupor), together with increasing breathlessness, ankle swelling, and even heart failure.

The vital outcome factor in all cases of bronchitis is whether or not progressive obstruction occurs to the passage of oxygen from the atmosphere to the blood. Such airflow obstruction, as it is called, occurs for two main reasons. First, persistent swelling of the linings of the air tubes from inflammation narrows them, and since many of the important smaller air tubes are no more than 0.04 in (1 mm) in internal caliber, obstruction by edema (accumulation of fluid) occurs very readily. Second, the total surface area available for the inward passage of oxygen and the outward passage of carbon dioxide becomes markedly reduced. Gas interchange in the lungs requires a very large surface area in the interface between the air and the blood. When large numbers of the tiny air sacs (alveoli) in the lungs break down to form larger spaces, a proportion of this surface is lost. This is what is called emphysema.

Monitoring lung function

The progress of lung damage in smokers can be accurately monitored by measuring the volume of air that can be expelled from the lungs in one second. This is called the forced expiratory volume (FEV), and the normal figure is about one gallon (3.5 liters). If the airways are narrowed, this volume will be reduced. In healthy nonsmokers, the FEV begins to drop from about the age of 20 at an average rate of 0.67 to 1.35 fluid ounces (0.02 to 0.04 liters) per year. In smokers with obstructive lung disease, the FEV drops two to three times faster than this. Treatment must therefore begin as soon as possible, starting with giving up smoking. Frequent acute attacks only worsen chronic bronchitis and make it harder to deal with. For these reasons preventive steps must also be taken to stem the progress of chronic bronchitis.

When people with mild to moderate airflow obstruction quit smoking, however, the rate of decline in FEV slows markedly and will eventually revert to that found in nonsmokers of the same age.

The rate of decline of lung function in smokers does, however, vary. A proportion of cigarette smokers with persistent (chronic) cough and sputum do not have breathlessness. In these people the tests of lung function do not reveal any detectable obstruction of airflow. Most smokers with productive coughs, however, develop significant narrowing of the lung airways.

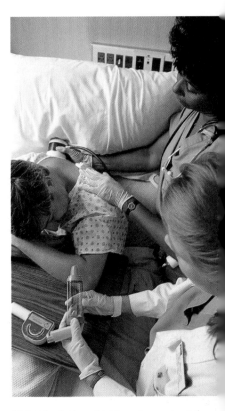

This physiotherapist is using a special electric device that emits vibrations that help loosen sputum in the patient.

Bruises

Q My son has bruised his shin badly while playing football. Is it possible that he could have damaged the bone in some way?

A Although the shinbone (tibia) is very near the surface of the skin, it is very strong and does not fracture easily. Nevertheless, if you are worried about him, you should seek medical help.

Q Is it true that children tend to bruise more easily than adults do?

A It often appears that children bruise more easily, but this is usually more a matter of their being more prone to accidents because of their nonstop activity. So it has more to do with the frequency of their falls and bumps than anything else. Children—and adults—who do seem to bruise more easily than other people should be checked by the family doctor. The elderly, because they lose the elasticity of their skin and because their capillaries (smaller blood vessels) become increasingly fragile, do bruise more easily than younger people.

Q I have noticed that my bruises take longer to fade than other people's. What is the reason for this?

A Four factors could be adding to the delay: your body's clearing mechanism may be slow in reaching the affected area; the bruising may be extensive and so take longer to clear anyway; or, if hematoma (small broken veins) occurs, you may need medical help. Or there is a slight possibility that you may have either a deficiency of vitamin C or of blood platelets, which will slow down the clotting process. You should see your doctor.

Q My neighbor, who is British, said that her doctor once gave her pills to help clear her bad bruising. Is this normal?

A In cases of severe bruising, some foreign doctors do sometimes prescribe pills, but this is not common practice in the US.

When the body receives a blow, bruising usually results. If this is severe, complications can arise; but most bruises will disappear within a few days.

A bruise can be recognized as a patch of dark or discolored skin anywhere on the head, face, trunk, or limbs and is the result of damage to the body's surface blood vessels. If the skin is unbroken, the bruise is known technically as a contusion; if it is more extensive, leading to the formation of a clotted lump of blood, it is called a hematoma.

Causes
If an accident occurs in which bruising takes place, the force may be sufficient to damage the small blood vessels—the capillaries—within the lining of the skin. If an even greater force is applied, small veins may be broken, and this could lead to the more massive form of bruising, which is called hematoma.

Bruising can happen as the result of virtually any sudden or violent contact or collision with a solid or blunt object. Sharp objects pierce the skin rather than bruise it; softer materials may leave no impression at all. A single bump will result in a single contusion; a car accident, for example, could cause multiple bruising, possibly all over the body, depending on the violence of the impact.

Symptoms
When a capillary breaks, blood will ooze out; it is this internal bleeding that gives the skin its familiar, dark red color. Any bluish tinge is partly caused by the red cells losing oxygen; the thickness of the skin can also distort the color.

The puffiness of bruises is caused by the release of the serous fluid (white blood cells and platelets) in the plasma. The platelets within the bruise initiate a process called coagulation (clotting), which limits the spread of the bruise and produces a substance, fibrin, that helps plug the leaking blood vessels.

A bruise will take between three and six days to clear, changing from reddish blue to greenish blue, and then to yellow. It then slowly fades. These color changes arise from the body's efforts to reclaim the blood that has leaked into the tissues, and it is this process that causes the bruise to fade.

Treatment
Small bruises with no break in the skin are best left to heal on their own. The only exception is where the bruise is under a toe- or fingernail, a condition called subungeral hematoma, for which

medical advice should be sought, because the end bone (the terminal phalanx) under the bruised nail may be broken. If the blood is released from under the nail, this will relieve pain and reduce the risk of infection. It will also help prevent the nail from turning black.

When bruises occur along with open wounds or lie over bony structures such as the skull, ribs, arms, and legs, they may conceal a fracture. In the case of bruises to the face and scalp especially, it is always advisable to consult the doctor to rule out the possibility of any underlying fracture or other damage.

First aid, in the form of gentle compression to the injury, using either an ice pack or a cloth soaked in cold water, will limit the pain and swelling if applied quickly. Painkillers such as acetaminophen will ease discomfort and help reduce bruising. Aspirin, which is an anticlotting agent, should be avoided as it can delay the healing process.

Larger bruises that result in hematoma should be seen by a doctor, who may decide to release the pressure of the blood in the swelling by simple surgery. This will deprive bacteria in the damaged tissue of any nourishment. Failure to treat boxer's hematoma can lead to the deformity cauliflower ear.

A bruised fingernail may cover a small broken bone, so it is always best to seek medical advice.

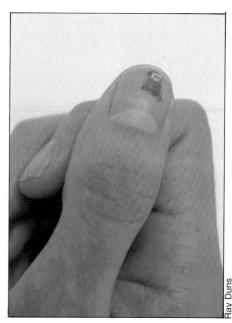

Ray Duns

Bunions

Wearing poorly made and badly shaped shoes could result in bunions—a painful foot deformity that may require surgery. But prevention is simple: wear comfortable, good-fitting shoes.

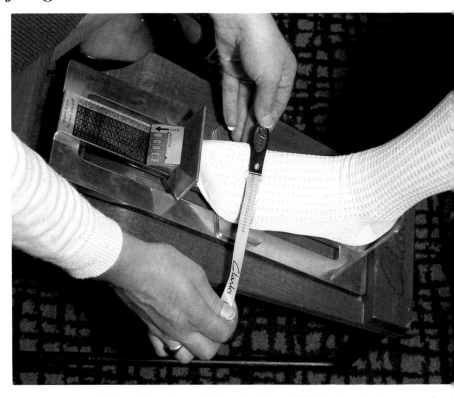

Having a child's feet properly measured an being careful to always buy well-fitting shoe insures against bunions.

Bunions are unsightly and can be painful, but they can usually be avoided. All that is required is just a little care in the choosing and fitting of shoes.

A bunion, which arises as a result of pressure, is an abnormal enlargement at the joint between the foot and the beginning of the big toe. All joints are surrounded by a capsule of fibrous tissue, and there may also be a bag of fluid, called a bursa, which cushions the movements of the various parts of the joint.

When the big toe joint gets swollen and inflamed, more fluid collects there and the ends of the bones may actually enlarge. Instead of the joint lying in a straight line, it is forced outward at a sharp angle. This puts pressure on the tissues between the bones and the shoe, resulting in the formation of a bunion.

The overlying skin may also become thickened and inflamed, and matters can be made worse by the fact that all this happens just where most shoes rub.

How bunions develop

This distortion of the big toe joint is usually caused by wearing shoes that are too tight for the toes. Women's shoes have traditionally been made narrower at the front than men's (although the anatom of male and female feet is exactly th same), so consequently women hav always tended to develop bunions mor frequently than men.

The trouble is increased by women shoes having higher heels. These forc the foot deep into the tight front of th shoe and put maximum pressure on th side of the big toe. If this sideways pre sure continues day after day, the big to joint is pushed out of place and becom deformed, leading to a condition calle hallux valgus.

When this arises, the big toe poin across to the other toes, while the fo bone under the skin leading to the b toe points outward. Once this state affairs is established, any further pressu from shoes will particularly fall on the b toe joint and cause a bunion to for there. At the other side of the foot, a si ilar deformity can arise, forming a sm bunion at the little toe joint.

Some people are born with a tenden to get hallux valgus and therefore a more likely to develop bunions. This may be because they have feet that are unusually broad in front so that off-the-rack shoes never fit properly. More rarely, the foot bone leading to the big toe may have started life abnormally and already be pointing outward.

Whatever the cause, once it is started, this deformity will tend to progress and not repair itself, even if no shoes at all are worn. This is because the tendons running to the toe bones become displaced. Instead of lying directly over the joint, they pull across to the inside. Then, every time the muscles contract to flex or extend the big toe—which happens at every step during walking—the pull of the tendons makes the condition worse.

Prevention and treatment
On the whole, shoe manufacturers are now well aware of public concern about foot deformities caused by badly fitting fashion shoes. As a result, wider shoes with lower heels are now available in more attractive styles. Shoes with very high heels and pointed toes that are worn regularly are bound to lead to problems, even in those fortunate enough to have narrow feet. Anyone who feels pain or notices redness of the skin on the outside of the big toe, should throw out their shoes immediately.

To see just how much room your feet take up, stand barefoot on a tape measure and compare the width of your toes with that allowed by your shoes; there is always a difference that represents the pressure that is being taken by your toes.

Due to the bowstring effect that is suffered by the tendons, treatment tends to be unsatisfactory. Wide-toed shoes are essential. A special pad may be worn between the big and index toes to try and correct the alignment of the big toe and reduce pressure on the bunion. In the end many women feel they have no alternative but to ask for an operation—but it is wise to remember that prevention is better than cure, so it is better to stop the problem from arising at all.

Complications
By itself a bunion is not a serious condition. Occasionally, however, it can become infected and require immediate treatment. The trouble may be caused by attempting to pare down the thickened skin as if it were a corn (see Corns)—this should never be done. Nor should a blister, which may have formed over a bunion, be opened. Once the skin is broken, infection is easily introduced and quickly spreads to the fluid of the bunion and then to the big toe joint. The joint will become even more swollen, red, and painful, and eventually pus may be discharged from it.

Treatment with antibiotics is then urgent to prevent any further spread of the infection and avoid septic destruction of the joint. If the sufferer is also in a generally run-down condition, the infection may take a long time to clear up completely.

As a long-term result of hallus valgus, the abnormal alignment of the big toe joint causes excessive wear and tear—and consequently arthritis. If the pain of the bunion has made a person walk in an abnormal way to compensate for the pain, there is a possibility that arthritis could also develop in other joints; this is a further complication that could have been avoided.

Surgery
Surgeons are reluctant to operate on bunions just for cosmetic reasons. And merely cutting out the bunion is never sufficient, because the trouble will only recur. A full operation must be performed to correct the deformity that actually removes the offending joint by cutting away the bone. Eventually this is replaced by strong bands of fibrous tissue that grow in its place—this will allow some degree of movement, but it will never be able to function like a joint.

After the operation, it takes some time before the patient can walk again without pain. For about three months any type of shoe will hurt, and most people do not feel they have received any benefit from the operation until after a period of about six months has elapsed. The patient should usually wear orthopedic shoes, at least during the recovery period.

How bunions are caused

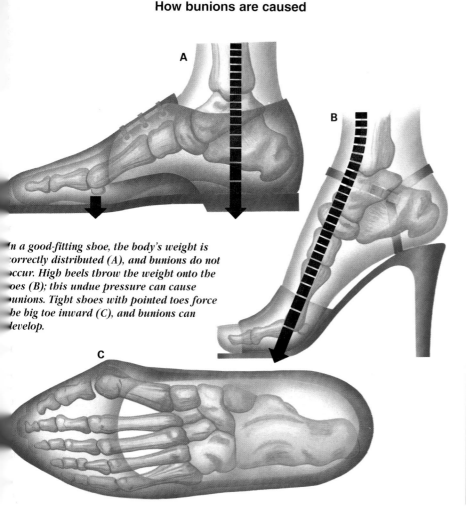

In a good-fitting shoe, the body's weight is correctly distributed (A), and bunions do not occur. High heels throw the weight onto the toes (B); this undue pressure can cause bunions. Tight shoes with pointed toes force the big toe inward (C), and bunions can develop.

Footnotes
- Do not start your children wearing shoes too early—let them go barefoot wherever it is safe to do so
- Discard shoes as soon as they are too small—even when they are favorites
- Have your child's feet regularly measured every two months
- Discourage teenage girls from wearing stiletto heels—especially if there are bunions in the family

Burns

Q My mother always believed in putting butter or olive oil on a burn she got while cooking. Are these any good as burn dressings?

A No, in fact she was doing more harm than good. Both oil and butter act as food for bacteria, which can develop and increase the risk of infecting the burn. For the same reason, you should never use ointments for first aid on burns; use clean, dry dressings instead.

Q How do I know when a burn is serious enough to call a doctor or to need hospital attention?

A If in any doubt, seek medical help immediately. This is especially vital for any of the following burns: on the face or genitals or over a joint; in the mouth or throat; if larger than 3 sq in (20 sq cm) or wet and oozing; if caused by electricity; if pain continues in spite of first aid; if on someone very young or old.

Q I read recently that it is not a good idea to drive a burn victim to the hospital yourself. Wouldn't this save time?

A Not if you were stopped by the police on the way—remember, you do not have the same traffic priority as an ambulance. Besides, your patient may need to be lying down and could vomit or lose consciousness as you drive, when you couldn't do anything to help.

Q Should I see a doctor if I get sunburned on vacation?

A If it is severe or combined with sunstroke, then the answer is yes. You should take special care to get used to the sun gradually if you are fair-skinned and not used to strong sunlight. Remember that you can even get sunburned in ice and snow on a mountain top, caused by the reflected ultraviolet radiation from the sun; also, if you are on a beach, the sun near the sea and sand is more intense than elsewhere. So take care in all situations in which you are exposed to strong sunlight.

The best way to deal with burns is to prevent them. But if an accident does happen, knowing what to do could mean the difference between life and death.

Countless people die or are severely injured every day through burns. Though it is generally assumed that the main cause is fire, burns can also result through touching hot objects or be caused by scalding, harsh friction, electric shock, or accidental contact with corrosive chemicals. The tragedy is even greater if you consider the ages of the victims. Understandably, very old people have the poorest chance of recovery from severe burns, but children are also vulnerable, especially toddlers, who do not understand the dangers involved in playing with fire.

Lesser burns

A burn is classified medically according to the depth that it reaches in the skin. There are three types: these are usually referred to as first-, second-, or third-degree burns. In the first group, also called superficial partial-thickness burns,

the epidermis (outer layer) of the skin is destroyed and the dermis (thicker, underlying tissues) may also be affected. But the hair follicles, sweat glands, and basic structure remain to form a basis for the growth of healthy new skin. The minor burns that happen in the kitchen or from sunburn (see Sunburn) fall into this category. The pain will stop within a couple of days, and the skin will soon recover. Sometimes a blister is formed; this protects the underlying wound from infection and should not be pricked. All the affected part needs is to be covered with a clean, dry dressing and allowed to heal.

More serious burns

In the second group—deep partial-thickness burns—all but the deepest cells, hair follicles, and glands are destroyed. With this type of burn, healing is slow and the new skin that is produced is likely to be rough and not as elastic as before.

Skin depths of first-, second-, and third-degree burns

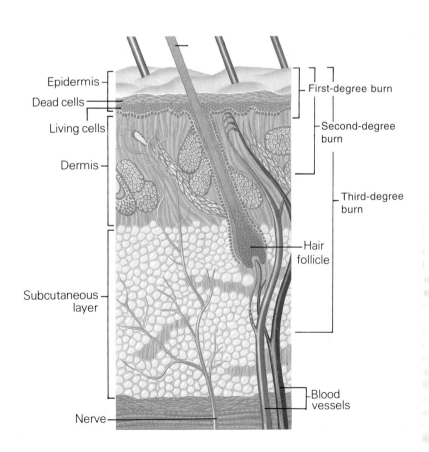

Treating burns

FIRST AID

The first treatment for every burn is to cool it off. For scalds, remove any clothing that has become hot from boiling fluid, fat, or steam. If the clothing has already cooled, however, do not remove it.

A chemical burn can be serious, so quickly remove any soaked clothing without touching the chemical yourself. Immediately wash away the chemical by flooding the area with water for at least 10 minutes.

An electrical burn requires fast action. Do not touch the victim until you have switched off the current. If this is impossible, call the power company or 911 immediately. Do not touch anything in contact with a downed wire.

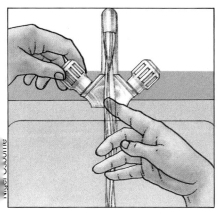

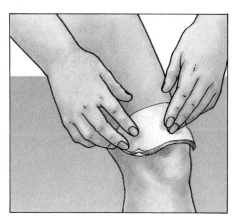

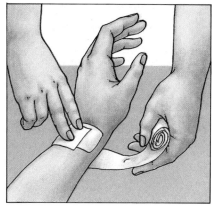

Always begin by cooling the burn. Major damage can be done by the heat from a burn penetrating deep into the body, and the application of cold water will help reduce this effect. A small part, like a fingertip or wrist, can be held under a running tap; a larger area should be plunged into a bucket or sink full of cold water.

Areas like the face or chest that cannot be kept underwater should be covered by a thick cloth soaked in cold water. If the cloth gets warm and dry, renew cold water and reapply. Continue cooling the burn for at least 10 minutes. This quickly relieves pain and reduces the formation of blisters. If much pain persists, repeat the procedure.

A large burn or a burn on the face should be covered with a nonfluffy dry dressing after cooling. Do not apply a lotion or ointment, and avoid touching the burn itself. Use the inside of a sterile surgical dressing or a clean handkerchief, handling it as little as possible. Cover with more folded padding and loosely bandage.

The most serious type of all is classified as a third-degree burn. Here the whole thickness burns, completely destroying the cellular structure of the skin; there is nothing from which the new skin can reform, unless it is at the very edges of the burn. In this event healing is extremely slow and uncertain. The whole area is more or less free of pain, however, because the nerve endings have been destroyed. But pain cannot be entirely absent, for at the edges of the burn there are likely to be some areas where nerve endings remain.

The loss of plasma (the colorless, liquid part of the blood) is one of the major problems with severe burns. What happens is that burns can form blisters that are filled with plasma that oozes out from the damaged blood vessels in the surrounding area. The blood cells are left behind. From this point of view, the area covered by a burn is more significant than the depth. Plasma, although it is

colorless and minus its cells, is still blood fluid, and a dramatic drop in its volume contributes to the condition called shock (see Shock). To make matters worse, the remaining blood in the body is now thicker, since its cells are concentrated in a smaller amount of plasma—this increases the difficulties of the heart, which may already be under stress.

Another problem is that a surface coating of plasma on the wound makes infection by bacteria much more likely. A great deal of protein is also lost, together with the plasma.

Hospital treatment

Hospital treatment is needed for all the deeper and more extensive burns. Relief of pain is, of course, important, but the primary concern is to combat shock.

The percentage of skin area to receive a burn is also an important factor in deciding the treatment to be given—for example, the back or front of the trunk

represents 18 percent of the whole surface of the body, while a hand represents one percent. A transfusion is likely to be needed when the burned area represents more than 15 percent of the total skin surface in an adult or more than 10 percent in a child. The fluid is generally plasma, but sometimes whole blood is included to replace red blood cells that have been destroyed.

Besides the transfusion, the patient's general condition must be closely watched, because the burned area will have lost much of its natural defense against bacteria. Not only does infection delay healing; it also increases the risk of disfigurement from scarring, and these scars may contract and interfere with the movement of any joint they overlie. Antibiotics (see Antibiotics) will be prescribed to combat any infection and thereby help in the healing process.

A partial-thickness burn is generally allowed to heal spontaneously, either by

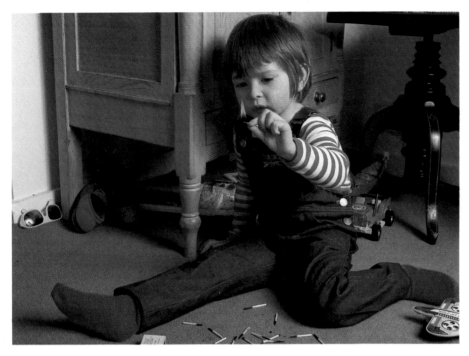

Young children are fascinated by fire and do not understand the dangers. Matches and other potential hazards should be kept out of their reach at all times.

being left exposed or being covered by a dressing. Healing may take between two and three months.

A full-thickness burn will not mend in this way, since the regenerating tissue has been destroyed. The dead material eventually separates off as dark, hard slough, leaving a raw area below. Frequently, it has to be helped off gently by the doctors and nurses, and a skin graft will be necessary to close up the wound.

When a skin graft is performed, small pieces of skin are removed from another part of the patient's body (usually from a place that is ordinarily covered by clothing). This healthy skin is implanted into the burned area and gradually grows to re-form a new skin surface. This process demands several months of skillful care, and it is especially important to insure that the grafted skin does not contract, which can affect the joint below.

Victims of severe burns may also need a high calorie diet containing extra iron and vitamins and also rich in protein to replace what has been lost in the plasma. Other organs, located far away from the original injury, may also have been damaged: the liver, stomach, intestines, gallbladder, and kidneys, for example. This can happen because shock following the injury reduces the blood supply to vital organs, causing damage that will not show immediately. These organs are kept under surveillance while the patient is in the hospital. Physiotherapy will be given

as soon as possible to maintain the health and fitness of undamaged limbs.

What to do in case of fire

If someone is trapped by a fire, cover your nose and mouth with a wet cloth. Reach the victim by crawling on the floor, where smoke is less dense. Guide or pull the victim out, and if he or she is choked by hot fumes, give artificial respiration. Victims may panic and run around beating at their clothes—actions that are likely to fan the flames. Try and stop this by getting the victim on the floor, with the burning area uppermost to allow flames to rise away from the body.

To extinguish flames, use water if possible; if not, smother the flames with thick material such as a rug, heavy towel, or coat. Throw this toward the victim's feet, thereby directing the flames away from the face. Press down gently to exclude air, but do not press any hot, smoldering cloth against the skin. Pull this away, but do not try and tear away any material sticking to the skin. Never roll the victim around; this would only expose different areas to the flames.

Other forms of treatment

When a burn is extensive, the risk of shock is high. To treat for shock, keep the victim lying down and loosen any tight clothing. Cover lightly. In the case of a burn, a cupful of water should be given, to be sipped every 15 minutes. Be reassuring and calm, but send for an ambulance immediately.

Do not try to remove any charred but cold material that may be sticking to the skin. Remove any jewelry, such as a ring,

Fire and burn prevention

Smoking Stub out cigarettes thoroughly in an ashtray. Do not throw cigarette stubs into a wastepaper basket. Do not smoke in bed or near inflammable material, for instance, in a garage

Cooking Light match before turning on gas tap. Never hang cloths over oven. Fill deep fryer no more than halfway and watch constantly; have large metal lid handy to smother flames in case of fire and keep fire blanket by cooker for the same purpose. Never put a hand in front of steam from kettle

Heating Have sturdy fireguards. Sweep chimneys regularly. Do not use paraffin or gasoline to light fires. Keep rugs away from fireplace. Ban toys from mantelpiece, and never place mirror on wall above fire. Insure oil heaters are firmly based. Never fill or carry them when lit

Clothes Beware of light cotton fabrics. Buy flameproof nightwear for children and old people

Wiring Replace frayed electric wires, loose connections, trailing leads. Fit correct fuses. Switch off to disconnect apparatus not in use, always pull out plug. Do not connect heaters or irons to lamp sockets

General planning Keep a fire extinguisher handy. Clear papers and rags from attic or under stairs

bracelet, or necklace, that could constrict the burned area, which may swell. Do not lance a blister, nor apply anything other than cold water. If there are no surgical dressings handy, use a clean handkerchief or towel. To insure maximum hygiene, handle the improvised dressing only by one corner. Let it fall open to unfold, and use the inside surface on the burn. Over this, place a padding of more folded material (another clean handkerchief or small towel) and secure with an improvised bandage, such as a necktie or panty hose.

If the face is burned, cut holes in the dressing to let your patient see. However badly swollen eyelids may keep the eye closed. Move the victim as little as possible, but be sure to keep a burned limb raised to reduce swelling—a large pillow or sling can be used. Reassure the victim as much as possible.

Burping

Q My husband's family all seem to have a burping problem. Can this run in families?

A Yes. If it is acceptable behavior in his family to burp, then there will seem no good reason to suppress this. However, it should be possible to persuade your husband to make the effort to control the habit if you want him to conform to the social norm. It may be simply a matter of reviewing his eating and drinking habits and keeping his mouth closed if he feels a burp coming on. It can be dispelled inside the mouth or reswallowed.

Q My brother is always burping and claims he can't help it. Why is he doing this?

A The most likely thing is he is swallowing air, although he may be unaware of this. If he has no other gastric symptoms, it is most unlikely that this is a medical problem. He is probably using his burps to call attention to himself.

Q My baby cries a lot after he has been fed. I spend ages trying to burp him, but nothing ever happens. Am I doing anything wrong?

A No. He's probably not getting up gas because he has not swallowed much air and there is nothing to bring up.

Q Does a good, loud burp have anything to do with the appreciation of a good meal?

A In American society, a burp is considered antisocial. In countries where excessive eating is a pleasure of life, and the stomach distension of a good meal can be relieved by burping, it can be seen as a compliment.

Q Why do men burp more than women?

A They don't—both sexes have an equal tendency to burp. However, men have always tended to be more overindulgent in food or beer, both of which tend to cause an excess of gas and burping.

Burping, or bringing up gas, is a normal reflex action in babies after a meal. Adults, however, can learn to control the response—if they so choose.

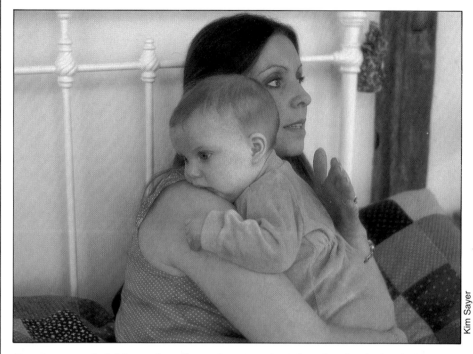

Kim Sayer

Burping—or belching—describes the involuntary reflex (backward flow) of gas from the stomach and out of the mouth. With every mouthful of food swallowed, some air is also taken down into the stomach. Babies swallow a lot of air as they suck in their milk; the actual amount varies with how well and hard the baby sucks and how much milk is available from the breast or bottle.

Adults often swallow excessive amounts of air, and this results in uncontrollable burps. Carbonated drinks contain an excess of dissolved gas, which is quickly released in the stomach—this can also cause burping, as can air swallowed to cool the taste of very hot food or to hide the taste of unpleasant food.

People who eat their meals too quickly and swallow a lot of air to help things go down are often prone to burping and sharp stomach pain.

How it happens

Once in the stomach, air can escape in two directions. It can pass on with the food into the small intestine (but this passage is closed immediately after a meal to insure food is adequately digested in the stomach before being allowed to progress down to the gut) or it can return back up the esophagus (the tube that extends from the throat to the stomach) to the mouth. This means any excessive

Burping is best done by placing the baby on your shoulder and firmly patting its back.

buildup of gas will put pressure on the valve at the stomach entrance, which is also closed to prevent food being regurgitated (thrown up).

As the stomach churns away, this pressure may suddenly get to be too much for the valve so that a burst of gas is released up the esophagus without warning. At the mouth, a late attempt to stop it merely increases the force of the explosion.

Prevention

Burping is a natural phenomenon, not a disease. Children are taught to control their burps, since the habit is considered antisocial. Eating more slowly and not swallowing too much air along with hot or spicy food will help.

In babies up to six months burping may cause concern. After being fed, the baby should not be put directly to bed. A few cuddles will be appreciated, and during this time the baby may burp a little naturally. Traditional methods of bringing up gas may be used if the baby appears uncomfortable. The favorite remedy is to place the baby over your shoulder and pat his or her back gently but firmly. Preparations designed to help eliminate gas, often containing a herb such as fennel, may help in some cases.

Bursitis

Q My husband, who is a construction worker, has a sore shoulder that the doctor says is bursitis. If he continues in his job, will it just get worse?

A The pressure and weight of carrying heavy materials over his shoulder has formed a bursa, which has become inflamed and swollen. Either your husband should change his technique for carrying heavy objects or he should wear a special pad under his coat, which will prevent all the weight being taken by one spot. Without these changes, working will make the situation worse, and the area will become even more painful and swollen.

Q My eight-year-old son has a swelling behind his knee. Could this be bursitis?

A Yes. This type of bursitis, which appears in children, is called semimembranosus bursitis. The cause is unknown; it is not likely that he could have brought it on in any way. Usually the condition disappears without treatment in a couple of weeks; during that time strenuous or prolonged exercise involving the knee is best avoided. It is not harmful or a sign of illness, so there is no need to worry.

Q Does a bursa ever burst like a blister does?

A The only bursa that bursts occurs when the cause of the bursitis is a bacterial infection; but this is rare. Common bursitis is not an abscess that grows in size until pus is discharged. In acute bursitis the cells lining the bursa are inflamed and overactive, so fluid is formed under pressure. The pain is relieved by a doctor aspirating the fluid with a needle.

Q I have only to do weeding for 10 or 20 minutes before both my knees swell up. Is this gardener's knee?

A Yes. For some unknown reason, the knees are particularly sensitive to bursitis and become inflamed easily. The only answer is to try various knee pads or avoid this type of gardening.

Now known to be a more complex process than formerly understood, this condition includes the disorder called the impingement syndrome and is very common in sports.

A bursa is a fluid-filled pouch formed in soft tissue, usually overlying a bone or joint. Bursitis is the inflammation of one of these sacs and is a common, and occasionally painful, condition requiring prompt treatment to prevent the inflammation from becoming acute or chronic.

There are two types of bursa. The most common, called anatomical bursas, occur on specific sites where tendons cross bones or joints. There are 15 such bursas around the knee joint alone. These usually pass unnoticed until they enlarge and bursitis develops.

The second type of bursa is one that arises purely as a result of repeated friction or injury to soft tissue overlying a bony surface. These are called adventitious bursas, and they may develop, for example, over the pelvic bone in the buttock from sitting on too hard a seat for several hours a day.

Both types of bursa act as shock absorbers and pressure pads, reducing the friction where tendons or ligaments move over bones. Only when the bursa

A typical prepatellar bursa (formerly called housemaid's knee). This can be avoided by simple preventive measures.

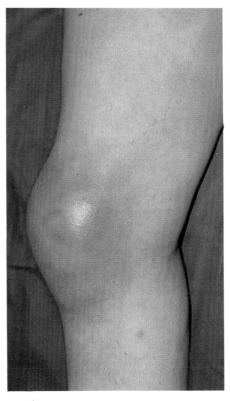

becomes chronically enlarged or acutely inflamed will bursitis develop. Prepatellar bursa, a condition that used to be called housemaid's knee and anatomically called the suprapatellar bursa, is caused by repeated pressure to the knee; any friction or injury causes the bursa to secrete fluid, resulting in the swelling.

Causes

Not all the causes of bursitis are always clear. Although it can affect both children and adults, some people are more likely to suffer than others.

Where friction causes the development of the bursa, the condition may be due to the way certain occupations or activities are carried out. Bursitis of the elbow, for instance, is common among students leaning on desks and miners crawling along tunnels. Porters sometimes develop bursitis at the neck from the pressure caused by carrying heavy boxes or baskets, as do construction workers from balancing loads of bricks. Weavers, who sit for long periods on hard loom seats, can develop bursitis on the buttocks; gardeners who work from a kneeling position are more likely to develop bursitis on the knees. However, the rubbing effect is not the complete explanation, since some people develop bursitis much more quickly than others.

In rarer cases bursitis can be caused by bacterial inflammation in the bursa or in a connecting joint. Tuberculosis was a common cause in the past. In some cases of rheumatoid arthritis, the bursa around a joint becomes inflamed; in rare cases gout may develop in a bursa. In bursitis of the elbow, which commonly occurs in older men, an identifiable cause rarely appears at all, and yet within a matter of hours a swelling the size of a hen's egg can appear.

Symptoms

In cases of acute bursitis, a swelling appears over a joint or bone. The swollen area is painful, tender to touch, and may feel hot and appear red; in severe cases movement is very painful. The fluid in acute bursitis is produced by the cells that line the wall of the sac. They produce a straw-colored fluid, often tinged with blood, since inflammation causes small blood vessels to leak. Where there is bacterial infection, this fluid becomes filled with bacteria and white blood cells to form pus, which may occasionally discharge. Chronic bursitis is caused by repeated attacks of acute bursitis or repeated injury causing swelling of a bursa. Slightly painful or even painless swelling may follow exercise or injury.

Bursitis is hardly ever dangerous. Bacterial spread, septicemia (blood poisoning), or spread of tuberculosis are rarely seen in these days of antibiotics. Untreated gout or rheumatoid arthritis may cause harmful inflammation elsewhere in the body, and chronic, unattended bursitis will eventually lead to wasting of the surrounding muscles, which in turn may weaken the joint.

Occupational hazards

Most of the former causes of bursitis in Western societies were occupation related. Health and safety regulations now, to a large extent, control the damage that may be done to the bodies of workers by pressure effects of this kind. The replacement of unskilled labor by machinery has also greatly reduced the incidence of most of the former types of bursitis.

These earlier, trade-related cases have now been replaced by a rising incidence of cases of sports-related conditions that are essentially self-inflicted. Formerly, sports were played largely for the pleasure of playing, rather than for the satisfactions of winning. Today competitive

pressures drive people, especially professional sportspeople, to make unprecedented demands on their bodies. Advances in orthopedics and sports medicine have shown that some of the conditions formerly described as bursitis involve a much greater complexity of causes than simply the production of excess fluid in bursas as a result of repeated pressure.

Impingement syndrome

The impingement syndrome is the current term for a group of conditions affecting various parts of the body, especially the shoulder, that were formerly described by a number of terms, including bursitis. These conditions are most commonly seen in people who practice sports involving throwing and swimming. What all these activities have in common is abnormally frequent impingement of one internal structure on another, especially when the arm is rotated outward and moved away from the body, and when it is moved repetitively in and above the horizontal plane.

Repetitive overhead use of the arm causes the tendons of the the rotator cuff to rub against the shoulder blade and its ligaments. The rotator cuff consists of the tendons of four adjacent muscles, blended with the capsule of the joint.

One of these muscles, the supraspinatus, becomes inflamed and weakened by repetitive use. When this happens, the rotator cuff is no longer able to depress the head of the upper arm bone (the humerus) into its shallow socket, and the more powerful deltoid (shoulder pad) muscle causes the head of the humerus to ride up, altering the way the joint works and making the situation worse. Considerable inflammation of tendons and bursas results, and inflamed tissue causes further impingement and damage.

Stages of the syndrome

The syndrome can be divided into three stages. The first resembles a simple bursitis, with inflammation and swelling from fluid production (edema) of the rotator cuff. The bursa lying under the process of the shoulder blade (the subachromial bursa) is commonly greatly swollen. In the second stage, pressure effects lead to an inadequate blood supply to the rotator cuff, and there is a progressive degeneration and scarring. The third stage involves a partial or complete tear.

Treatment

The treatment for acute bursitis should be supervised by a doctor, in case the cause is bacterial infection or another rarer cause. If the cause is unknown, or if the bursitis is due to rubbing, friction, or

A common site of bursitis

In the normal shoulder (below), the bursa stops the tendon from rubbing on the shoulder joint. If undue pressure is put on a shoulder, the bursa will become inflamed and sore (insert). This can be avoided by padding the area.

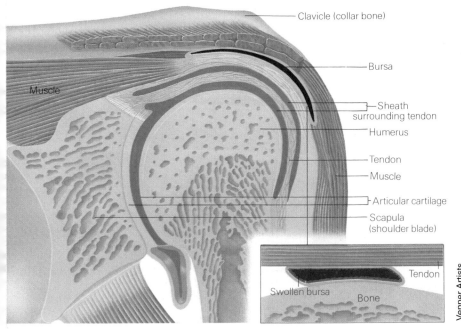

Clavicle (collar bone)
Bursa
Muscle
Sheath surrounding tendon
Humerus
Tendon
Muscle
Articular cartilage
Scapula (shoulder blade)
Swollen bursa
Bone
Tendon

Venner Artists

excess use, then resting the affected joint or area, with only passive exercise for the surrounding muscles, is the cure.

If there is pain, painkillers (see Painkillers) may be needed. Anti-inflammatory drugs, such as those used to treat arthritis, may reduce the amount of fluid secreted by the cells lining the bursa. Antibiotics will only be necessary if there is also a bacterial infection present.

A cold compress or ice pack may help reduce the inflammation. Cool a glycerin or crushed-ice-filled polyethylene bag in the refrigerator. Mold the cold bag to the contours of the skin, checking that it is not so cold as to irritate the affected area. Then bandage lightly with a stretch bandage. Keep this on for half an hour before removing. If this treatment provides relief, repeat the treatment as often as possible, up to once every four hours, until the condition improves.

If the condition does not improve within two or three days, the doctor may aspirate (drain) the bursa, using a hypodermic needle. First a local anesthetic is applied, then the needle is inserted deep into the bursa. Some of the fluid is then sent to a hospital laboratory to be checked for the presence of bacteria.

Avid gardeners can avoid the risk of bursitis by using a special kneeling pad for tasks such as weeding.

The doctor might also inject hydrocortisone, a steroid drug that has an anti-inflammatory effect, into the bursa. Once drained, the bursa is bandaged firmly. This treatment may have to be repeated a number of times before the effect becomes permanent.

Surgical removal

The surgeon cuts away as much of the fluid-forming sac as possible and clears out the accumulated clumps of clotted protein. This surgical removal of the bursa is usually successful, although in a small minority of cases the bursa will form again in a few weeks.

As far as treatment of the impingement syndrome is concerned, the first stage involves strict rest from the activity that has caused it. It may be necessary to avoid all overhead movement of the arm for a period. Drugs to control inflammation and fluid production are given. In severe cases it may be necessary to inject steroids directly into the subachromial bursa. Once the pain has been relieved an active physical therapy program is needed to restore full movement and to strengthen the muscles that control the rotator cuff.

There are various surgical procedures that can be used to reduce the pressure in the area under the shoulder blade (the subachromial space). This may involve

removing part of the shoulder blade and part of the whole bursa.

Outlook

Pain and difficulty on movement is to be expected in cases of acute bursitis, and with treatment, this condition usually clears completely within a week or 10 days. If the cause is bacterial inflammation, the likelihood of recurrence is very rare indeed.

With chronic bursitis, the condition usually only recurs if the stimulus of rubbing or friction is repeated. For this reason, taking preventive measures is very important. Thick clothing or padding of areas exposed to pressure is essential. Adequate cushioning on seating helps prevent buttock bursas and, to prevent the most common bursitis, prepatellar, knee pads are absolutely essential for all jobs such as floor laying or gardening. Anyone who develops inflammation in the Achilles tendon of the ankle—achillobursitis—should be sure to avoid violent exercise.

In the case of the impingement syndrome, the outlook depends on the stage at which proper treatment is given. If the condition has been neglected in the early stages, it may be necessary for the athlete to avoid all overhead activities permanently. Sometimes pain persists even when this is done.

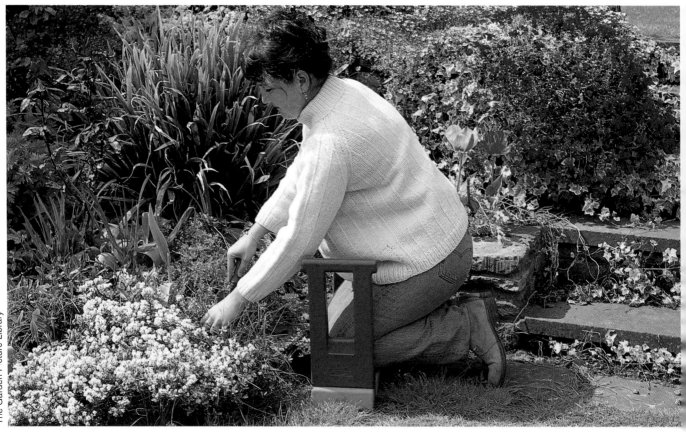

Caesarean birth

Q I was so bitterly disappointed at not giving birth naturally, that I cannot help feeling like a failure. I have been real depressed and at times find it hard to feel affection for the baby. How can I get over this?

A First, having a Caesarean is not a failure on your part. You did your best, and the operation was a necessity beyond your control. Women who have Caesareans should be applauded for their success in coping with their recovery and a tiny baby as well. It is natural to be depressed following any major operation, especially a Caesarean, when the body is undergoing hormonal changes as well as healing. Some women are temporarily depressed following natural childbirth, too, because of this upset in hormones.

It is also understandable not to feel affection for the baby all the time when you are tired and probably have some discomfort. Talk things over with your doctor. You could also try talking to other new mothers near you, who will understand and sympathize with your feelings.

Q If my sister has had one Caesarean birth, will she have to have another with her next baby?

A It depends on why the operation was performed. For example, if she has a normal-sized pelvis, and the operation was performed because the baby was distressed and there was no progress in labor, it is still possible for another pregnancy to result in a vaginal delivery.

Q I have had two children, both born by Caesarean section, and I would like to have a third child. Is there a limit to how many Caesareans I can have before it becomes risky?

A There is no absolute limit to the number of Caesarean births a woman can have. Each individual case is assessed by the obstetrician. With a third pregnancy, it is possible that he or she may advise early admission and early delivery to prevent strain.

A Caesarean is a safe, speedy operation that is performed when a natural delivery is not possible or desired.

A Caesarean birth means that the baby is born through a surgical incision made in the mother's abdominal wall and uterus (womb). It may be performed either as an emergency, when the life and health of the mother or baby are at stake, or be planned in advance because the doctors know that natural birth is impossible or unsafe in the particular circumstances.

A planned Caesarean

Although it depends on the reason for the operation, most women who are having a planned Caesarean section enter the hospital when they are 38 weeks pregnant or before. Tests will make sure the baby is mature enough to be delivered without being harmed.

The night before the operation, a routine examination of the mother will be performed, the pubic area shaved, and an enema given to clear her intestine. Blood samples will be taken in advance for grouping and cross-matching in case a blood transfusion should be needed.

If a general anesthetic is to be used, the mother will be given nothing to eat or drink after midnight the night before the operation. However, many hospitals do a Caesarean section under epidural anesthesia (an anesthetic inserted into the epidural space just in front of the spinal cord, which numbs the area below). With

an epidural, the mother can hold her baby immediately after birth, and the father may be allowed to watch the birth. Therefore, if a woman knows she needs to have a Caesarean section, she should ask about an epidural if she wants to be aware of what is happening.

Emergency Caesareans

Although "emergency Caesarean" sounds like a life-or-death situation, it rarely is. Once in the operating room, medical experts frequently safely perform the operation and deliver the baby in just five to seven minutes.

Problems with the baby are picked up at an early stage on a machine called a fetal monitor. This is done either by means of electronic recordings of the fetal heart via a tiny clip attached to the baby's scalp or by microphones attached to the mother's abdomen.

If a problem is detected, preparations for the operation are hasty. An intravenous infusion (drip) will be set up. Fluids are essential for the prevention of shock, and extra blood may be required through a blood transfusion. The abdo-

Approximately 25 to 30 percent of births in the United States are by Caesarean section, but each birth remains a unique event for parents and medical staff alike.

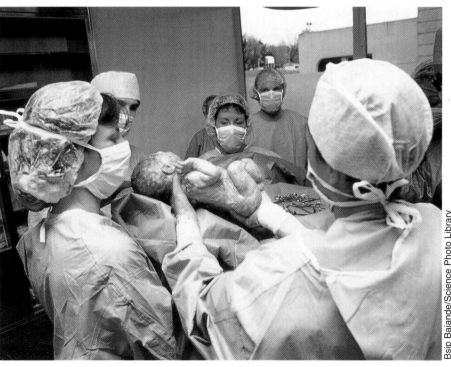

Bsip Bajande/Science Photo Library

Reasons for an emergency Caesarean

Before labor, as a result of unexpected bleeding due to:
- separation of placenta from uterine (womb) wall
- placenta previa—the placenta has grown across the neck of the womb (cervix). The cervix opens up prior to labor, and the placenta starts to detach, with bleeding

The baby is suffering from:
- fetal distress—this shows up on the monitor. The baby's heartbeat may slow and become irregular
- lack of oxygen due to prolapse of the umbilical cord. The cord comes out through the vagina ahead of the baby. The change in temperature makes the blood vessels in the cord contract, cutting off the blood supply that carries oxygen from mother to baby
- pressure on the cord, which stops oxygen being carried to the baby

During labor, due to the mother's exhaustion because of:
- poor or no progress in labor
- high blood pressure—the mother may be prone to this condition, or it may have been caused by health difficulties during pregnancy
- failed induction of labor. If labor is started artificially by breaking the water and giving a drug that stimulates contractions, and this fails, the operation is necessary to avoid harm to mother and baby
- mother has active genital herpes, and passage of baby through the birth canal would expose him or her to a potentially fatal infection

Why a planned Caesarean may be necessary:

- the outlet of the pelvis is smaller than the baby's head
- there are pelvic abnormalities of that would prevent natural birth
- there is a disease that would endanger the mother's life if she gave birth naturally, such as a heart or lung disease
- the mother has diabetes. However, more is now known about this, and diabetic mothers can often have their babies naturally
- there has been a previous Caesarean section and a second may be required
- breech presentation—the baby is positioned feet or bottom first, which can prolong labor

How a Caesarean delivery is performed

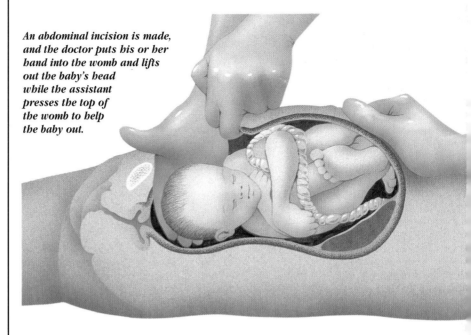

An abdominal incision is made, and the doctor puts his or her hand into the womb and lifts out the baby's head while the assistant presses the top of the womb to help the baby out.

men and pubic area are quickly prepared by shaving before the anesthetic is given.

With a general anesthetic, the mother-to-be will now be unconscious. A rubber tube is placed in her bladder to empty it before the operation. The nurse-midwife checks the fetal heart on the monitor at regular intervals before the surgery begins. In this type of emergency situation, the father may not be permitted in the operating room in case it upsets him, but he is usually allowed to sit nearby in a waiting room.

The operation

Nowadays most obstetricians—doctors who specialize in pregnancy and birth—make the incision in the lower part of the abdomen on the bikini line so that a scar will not show. Forceps are inserted to hold back the layers of tissue. The lower segment of the womb is exposed and the internal incision is widened. The doctor puts his or her hand into the womb to lift out the baby's head. (Forceps may be used to deliver the head.) The assistant presses the top of the womb to push the baby out. The placenta is delivered, and the mother is given a drug to contract the womb. The abdomen is then stitched.

Meanwhile the baby is given immediately to the pediatrician (baby doctor), who is always present to check the newborn. The suddenness of the birth can cause the baby some shock, and it can take a few minutes for him or her to respond normally. It may take a while for the breathing to become regular and for the heart rate to steady. This is normal and need not cause concern. Sometimes the

baby can be lethargic because of the anesthetic given to the mother, and he or she may need drugs to counteract the effects.

Most babies are put into incubators to warm up and to be observed while the mother comes around from the anesthetic. If all is well, mother and baby can go back to the ward and both parents may hold and cuddle the baby.

Care of the mother

With a general anesthetic, it may be several hours before the mother really feels she knows where she is. Indeed it is common for women to forget having seen their babies when they were first shown them by the doctor.

The abdomen is very tender for several days, and it is difficult to move at first. A drip-feed into a vein may have been put in place after the operation, and it will stay in until the digestive system is working properly, which may take several days. It may also take the mother time to urinate easily. But pain relief is always available and may be necessary to begin with. The mother can breast-feed her baby before she takes pain-relief injections, so that there is a minimal drug effect on the baby.

Tiredness eases as time passes, but feeding can be exhausting to start with. If a mother does not want her baby to have formula milk, she can request breast milk from the milk bank if it is available. Otherwise she can express her own milk to allow her extra sleep.

Day two

Getting up and walking on the second day is advised because of the risk of blood clots in the legs. The mother will be encouraged to get up for a few minutes even on the first day. She should not be surprised if she feels exhausted.

The tube in the bladder and the drip will be removed if all is well. Sometimes there is a small drainage tube in the wound, but this is usually taken out after 48 hours. Most hospitals have visiting physiotherapists who may suggest chest exercises to prevent infection and static blood flow due to inactivity. The mother may still want pain relief, but this need will soon pass.

Day three

The mother will now have more energy and be feeling less tired when she gets up. She may have a bath with help. If there is a problem going to the bathroom, a suppository—a pill inserted in the rectum—may be given (see Suppositories). This helps relieve the distention and discomfort often felt after an operation on the abdomen. The clips or sutures are usually taken out on the sixth day, but this will be done on an outpatient basis after discharge at four days.

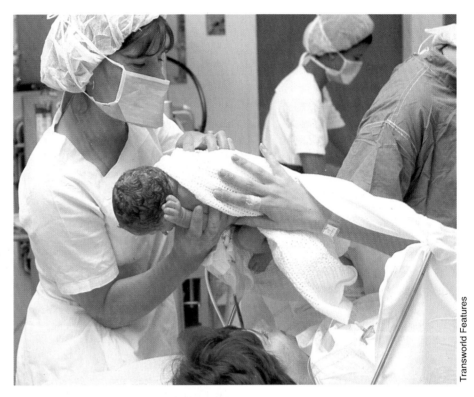

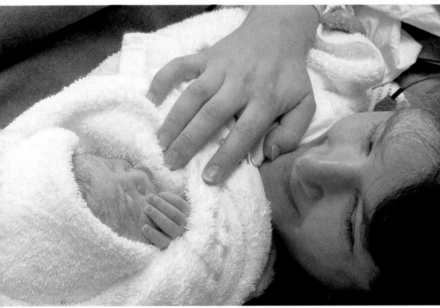

A woman can have an epidural anesthetic for a Caesarean and be conscious during the birth of her baby. She is handed the child immediately after the birth (above) and is able to hold and cuddle the infant (left); even while the doctor stitches her incision, she feels no pain or discomfort.

Long-term effects

A woman may find that it is several months before she feels really well, and this is quite natural. She may find the wound from the operation tender and sore for some weeks, and bending and lifting may be difficult. This all improves with time. Planning for help at home is essential for at least a few weeks. The baby's father may be able to do more around the home than usual during this time, or a relative might come to stay.

Postnatal exercises may be too uncomfortable to do at first, but they can be done later. Sometimes it takes a bit of time to urinate for a few weeks due to loss of bladder tone, which will return.

Sexual intercourse can be uncomfortable while the wound is still sore, but discomfort can also be due to the tenderness of the internal pelvic organs, which have been handled during the operation. If discomfort is prolonged, advice should be sought from the doctor or the hospital.

Emotional problems

Many women feel they have failed by not having a natural birth. But having a

Caesarean section and coping with a new baby is far from failing. Usually the excitement of the new baby overrides the fact that there was a major operation. However, partners and relatives need to remember that the mother needs special help, care, and attention.

If there were complications and the mother was separated from the baby after the operation, delayed early contact may mean that she finds it harder to feel immediate maternal feelings. This is especially so if she feels sore and in temporary pain and discomfort. It is natural not to feel immediately close to the baby after a Caesarean section, and temporary depression is perfectly normal too. Only when these feelings continue for a long time will expert help be needed.

Many women worry about their operation scar. It is permanent, but it fades slightly with time. If the incision was made at the bikini line, it will be covered by underpants and will not be noticeable. In the rare cases where it may be necessary, a woman can have the scar removed by plastic surgery, but she should not do this if she intends to have more children, in case a future delivery should result in another Caesarean.

Calcium

Calcium is essential to the human body—and in amounts that are finely balanced so that we have neither too much nor too little. This balance can sometimes be upset, but treatment will correct it.

Q I have heard that too much calcium in the body is harmful. Could this happen to me if I ate too much in my food?

A No. The body regulates how much calcium is required through the intestine. It absorbs the correct amount of calcium from your blood, provided you eat an adequate diet. Excess calcium is passed out in the urine. However, taking excessive amounts of vitamin D pills can upset the system. If the absorption system goes wrong, it can lead to kidney stones. A low calcium diet helps to avoid this.

Q I am pregnant. Do I need calcium tablets to insure that my baby develops healthy bones and will have strong teeth?

A No, not unless your diet is lacking in protein-rich food and fruit and vegetables. The intestine compensates for you and your baby's requirements and will absorb more calcium from your food as necessary. However, it will do you no harm to drink some extra milk.

Q My grandmother, who is in her sixties, recently broke her arm in a minor accident. She believes that her bones have weakened since menopause. Is this possible?

A Yes. The estrogen present in women before menopause helps to build up calcium in the bones. After menopause, osteoporosis (a thinning of the bones) may set in, particularly in those who are not eating properly, so make sure that your grandmother has an adequate diet, especially if she lives alone and does not want to cook just for herself. Treatment with hormone replacements, calcium, and vitamin D will also produce great improvements.

Q How much milk should my three-year-old drink?

A Three glasses of milk contain half a gram of calcium—an adequate daily intake for a one- to nine-year-old. And since calcium is present in other foods, a good diet will easily provide enough calcium.

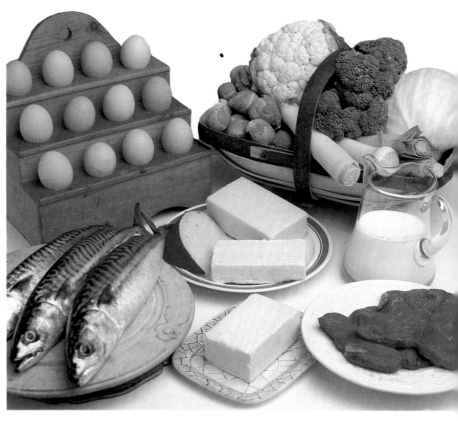

People need calcium throughout their lives to insure healthy bones and teeth; that is why a balanced diet is so important. Calcium-rich foods include milk, cheese, eggs, meat, fish, and vegetables.

Bones and teeth contain a large proportion of calcium. Calcium crystals form solid building blocks that are held together by a fibrous network; the result is a strong resilient material for supporting your body—the bones. However, calcium is not permanently located in the bones, for it can be mobilized to help maintain the correct levels in the body tissues elsewhere.

Small amounts of calcium also regulate the impulses from the nerves in the brain. Similarly they influence muscle contraction. Blood clotting also relies on a set amount of calcium in the blood.

Calcium balance

We absorb calcium from our food, and it passes, via the intestine, into the bloodstream. Some is lost in the urine. But some is stored in the bones or reabsorbed into the bloodstream.

To maintain a balanced level of calcium in the blood, the body has an elaborate control system. This is located in the parathyroid glands (see Parathyroid glands) in the neck. Their product—parathyroid hormone (PTH)—acts on the bones and kidneys to release more calcium and also to decrease loss in the urine.

When calcium levels are low, more PTH is passed into the bloodstream. When the levels are high, less PTH is sent out, and so a constant balance is maintained. Vitamin D is also essential for maintaining the balance of calcium. Without it, calcium cannot be absorbed from food. It also acts with PTH to release calcium from the bones.

Excessive calcium

If there is too much calcium in the body, symptoms such as vomiting and stomach pains develop. Even more seriously, excess calcium may be deposited in the kidneys and form renal stones. (Renal stones are usually excreted naturally without an operation, but this is painful.) Too much calcium could be the result of a parathyroid tumor secreting uncontrolled amounts of PTH. Alternatively it could simply mean that the sufferer had taken too many vitamin D pills.

In an emergency, calcium levels can be reduced by phosphate injections or pills. A parathyroid tumor needs surgery. If the cause is too many vitamin pills, the person must stop taking them.

A lack of calcium

If there is too little calcium, a condition called tetany occurs. The term describes spasms of the muscles, especially in the hands, feet, and larynx. A common cause of tetany is hysterical overbreathing, triggered by fear or emotion, which results in a chemical change that temporarily reduces available blood calcium. As the hysteria passes away naturally, the body returns to normal.

If the parathyroid glands have to be removed, to treat a parathyroid tumor, for example, PTH levels can suddenly drop and cause tetany. This can be successfully treated by giving calcium through a vein and oral vitamin D.

In addition to tetany, low calcium can produce abnormal blood clotting and unbalanced heart rhythms. However, the muscle spasms always reveal themselves first, and treatment prevents the other problems from developing. If low calcium levels are left untreated for months, other symptoms occur. The loss of calci-

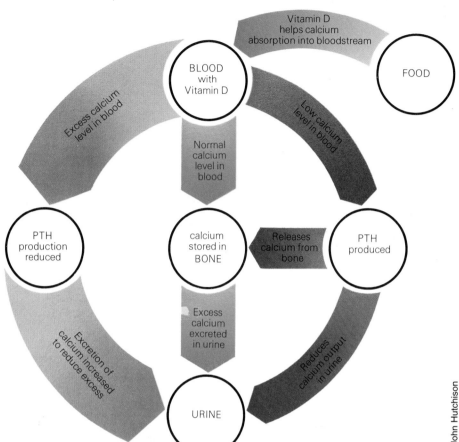

How the body maintains a normal calcium balance

Vitamin D helps calcium absorption into bloodstream

BLOOD with Vitamin D

FOOD

Excess calcium level in blood

Low calcium level in blood

Normal calcium level in blood

PTH production reduced

calcium stored in BONE

Releases calcium from bone

PTH produced

Excretion of calcium increased to reduce excess

Excess calcium excreted in urine

Reduces calcium output in urine

URINE

John Hutchison

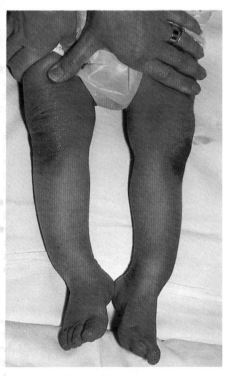

This child has rickets, a bone condition caused by calcium and vitamin D deficiency: the leg bones are soft and the legs bow outward.

um from the bones causes rickets (which results in bone deformities; see Rickets) in children, and osteoporosis (thinning bones) in elderly people. With these conditions, bones become weakened.

Rickets still occurs even today and can be helped by extra vitamin D. Many elderly people suffer from osteoporosis, partly as a result of living on a poor diet, such as tea, bread, and jam—food with very few vitamins. These people will benefit from additional calcium, but their diet should be improved generally.

The hormone calcitonin, given in pill form, is helpful to patients with osteoporosis, since it causes calcium to be deposited in the bones. Another disease of old age, Paget's disease, which has symptoms of thickened but weak bones, will also respond to calcitonin tablets.

Poor absorption of calcium is not a common problem. Intestinal disease can prevent vitamin D, and hence calcium, from being absorbed from food. Kidney disease patients are living longer due to improved treatment, but they tend to develop rickets. This is because vitamin D has to be stimulated by the kidneys to do its job. Kidney patients can be treated with extra vitamin D, however.

Vitamin D is necessary for calcium to be absorbed from food into the bloodstream. The level of calcium in blood is controlled by PTH (parathyroid hormone), which will be low if there is a lack of vitamin D. A lack of calcium in the blood causes PTH to be produced, and this encourages reduction of calcium stored in bones. Excess calcium in the blood reduces PTH production and results in calcium being excreted.

Mother and baby

If a woman is pregnant or breast-feeding, her body loses a lot of calcium and vitamin D to the baby. But her intestine compensates for this by absorbing more calcium and vitamin D from the food she eats. Provided a pregnant woman eats a balanced diet, there is usually no need for her to take calcium supplements.

If a mother is bottle-feeding the baby, great care should be taken to make up the formula milk according to the instructions on the package so that there will be no calcium problem. Vitamin supplements are normally added to babies' formula milks. Breast-fed babies are protected from a low calcium level by mother's milk and by vitamin D supplements, given in liquid drop form.

Calipers and braces

Q My brother says the doctor wants to fit him with a caliper because of an injured knee he got from a football injury. Will he always have to wear it?

A Probably not. Calipers, or braces, are often given as a temporary treatment for sports injuries, especially ones to the knees and ankles. When the device has done its job—usually a question of relieving strain so that the body can heal itself more efficiently—it need not be worn again.

Q If my husband has to have a caliper fitted to his leg in order to help him walk after his present attack of rheumatoid arthritis, will it make the leg weaker than ever?

A In this case, as in many others, the reason for wearing a caliper is to reduce the pain of walking, caused by excessive pressure on the ankle joint. If he didn't have the caliper, he would almost certainly walk much less, if at all. So by enabling him to give his weak limb extra use, it should improve his condition in the long run.

Q I've heard that some stroke patients can be fitted with a caliper to help them walk. My husband has had a stroke, and I think he might benefit from one, but will it make a terrible banging noise around the house?

A Most modern calipers have either no moving parts or very few, and therefore do not make noise. If a caliper does have joints, excessive wear may cause some noise, but this is easy enough to remedy by repairing or replacing.

Q Can a person take a caliper off in bed?

A Generally yes, unless it has been given for a certain serious hip problem.

Q My baby has spina bifida. Will he always need a caliper?

A Yes. But at least he will be able to move around and not be confined to a wheelchair.

Great advances have been made in the development of devices that either support or help parts of the body that have been damaged by disease or injury, giving wearers increased mobility and comfort.

Caliper, *brace*, and *splint* are all terms used to describe the same thing: a device for supporting or helping some part of the body that has lost its strength or the ability to work properly. This loss of strength or function can stem from a variety of causes.

The term *caliper* tends to mean a device for supporting the leg, but it may be used generally, as are the other words. Doctors will frequently use other technical terms for these devices, such as *appliances*, *orthotic devices*, or *orthoses* (in the singular, *orthosis*).

One name that should not be heard in connection with this subject is *leg iron*.

The term is no longer encouraged, because it is not a fair (or positive) description of equipment that, although superbly strong and supportive, is in some cases surprisingly flexible and comfortable. This is because, nowadays, calipers and braces are never made of iron. A variety of modern materials goes into their construction, although they are primarily made of steel and plastic, a combination that insures they are both lightweight and strong.

This young girl has spina bifida. She has been fitted with leg braces, which she is learning to use with the aid of crutches.

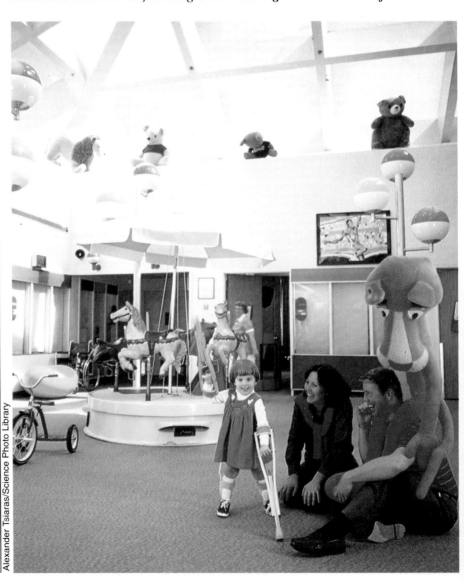

General uses

The word *caliper* usually means a device for supporting the body from the hips downward. A brace is generally understood to be worn around other parts of the body, such as the neck, spine, forearm, wrist, and fingers. In addition to simply supporting or assisting limbs, braces and calipers are prescribed to change the shape of deformed parts of the body, to increase body temperature, and to protect parts of the body.

Supply of calipers and braces

Any instruments used to support parts of the body must be carefully manufactured, and high standards and specifications must be adhered to. Each device must be tailored to an individual's measurements and needs according to the doctor's prescription, and this is an expensive process.

Many hospitals now have specialists who are trained in the precise fitting of splints, braces, calipers, and foot supports. This practice is called orthotics and has been increasingly helpful for arthritis patients. Also important is the training, given to the patient by a physiotherapist or occupational therapist, in how to put the brace on or take it off and in how to use it to full advantage.

Calipers

One of the most common types of caliper is called the ankle foot orthosis, or AFO. It will often be given to the patient who, after a stroke, has the tendency to drag his or her toes when walking (foot drop), as a result of losing proper use of the ankle joint.

The device consists of two steel rods carefully shaped to follow the outline of the shin and prevent rubbing on the rounded bone that sticks out at the ankle. The general framework is of specially molded polypropylene (nylon or plastic) sheeting. A clever refinement of the appliance is called functional electronic stimulation. This uses a miniature electronic stimulator in the heel to provoke a spasm in the relevant nerve thereby making the ankle move.

The KAFO

The knee ankle foot orthosis (KAFO) is otherwise called the long leg brace. The number of people who need it as a result of paralysis caused by polio (a nerve infection) or knee joint disorders are much fewer than they were in previous times. This is because vaccination has almost eliminated polio, and knee problems are usually treated successfully by operating. But the KAFO's use for two conditions, strokes and spina bifida, is sadly on the increase. The first causes various degrees

of paralysis over several areas of the body, including the legs. The second, a defect in the development of the baby's spine while the fetus is developing in the mother's womb, gives flailing legs and sometimes complete loss of feeling in the limbs.

The KAFO usually consists of steel rods that can move at the same time as the knee and ankle, attached to the leg with steel bands and leather straps. The knee joint often has a lock that allows the patient to sit down comfortably, with fully bent knees, but which automatically relocks for walking.

KAFOs are increasingly available in the new, plastic materials, which improve their appearance. In many cases they may be worn with ordinary styles of shoes, which increases the wearer's feeling of self-confidence.

The HKAFO

This stands for the hip knee ankle foot orthosis, which supports the whole of the lower half of the body. It is attached with leather straps around the chest and just below the buttocks, and has joints at the hip, knee, and ankle.

It is a major contraption, but to those faced with wearing it—particularly children with severe spina bifida—the device means, at least, the ability to move around more freely and not be confined to a wheelchair.

Surgical boots and shoes

These are all-too-common orthotic devices, and there is a simple reason for this: rheumatoid arthritis. This widespread disease causes pain, swelling, and stiffening of the joints, and as the human foot contains more than 20 joints, it is not surprising that rheumatoid arthritis sufferers have problems with their feet. There are also, of course, many other conditions that call for the use of surgical boots or shoes.

Special shoes are available in many forms, ranging from simple shoe adaptations (like a raised heel or modified areas of ground contact for the sole) to special inserts for easing pressure, or a heel cup to control a minor deformity of the ankle. There are also special boots built entirely to suit an individual's particular needs, and, of course, some degree of adaptation of shoes is usually required when calipers are fitted.

Back supports

Probably the most common type of brace worn on any other part of the body is the back support, prescribed for pain in the region of the lower back. It is made of fabric, with elastic sections and leather or webbing straps, and sometimes it has strong steel reinforcing "bones." Other

appliances that may be used for deformities and other problems of the back and neck include the Milwaukee brace; the Knight, or Chair, back brace; and the Williams brace.

Devices especially for the neck are usually called cervical collars. Their purposes are to support the spine as it runs through this part of the body and to control the direction in which the head is pointing.

Wrist and arm appliances

One of the most ingenious appliances for the hand is the wrist flexor splint, which allows movement to take place in otherwise paralyzed fingers and thumbs by transferring power from the wrist. There are also devices for straightening and bending the arms and several specialized pieces of equipment for correcting contractures of the digits and severe stiffness of the fingers.

The future

Calipers and braces have progressed enormously in design and appearance over the last decade, and there is no reason why they should not continue to do so in the future. The aim, as always, will be for greater improvements in strength, lightness, and reliability, and by making them compact, to allow theses devices to be hidden or disguised whenever possible. All of these factors will improve the quality of the treatment and the lives of those who have to wear them.

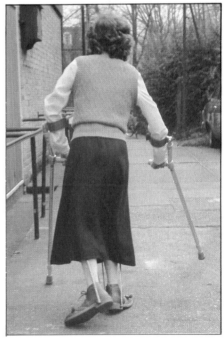
Henry Grant

The hip knee ankle foot orthosis supports the whole of the lower half of the body and has joints at hip, knee, and ankle.

Cancer

Q My brother-in-law has had a lot of X rays recently. Can these cause cancer?

A The risk of developing cancer from X rays is so small as to be insignificant. Doctors are, however, aware of this risk and will only advise you to have an X ray if they feel that it is absolutely necessary. The risk of not having the X ray is greater than the risk of having it.

Q Can cancer cells become resistant to the effects of cytotoxic drugs that are supposed to poison them?

A Unfortunately they can. The exact reasons for this are uncertain, but after a while a cancer cell will find ways of reproducing itself despite the presence of the cytotoxic drug, and the treatment must then be changed.

Q I have heard that interferon might cure many kinds of cancer. Is this true?

A Interferons are proteins produced by the body in response to viral infections. Certain interferons show definite promise against many viral diseases, but they have yielded only mixed results against cancers. They are a little promising against malignant melanoma and kidney cell cancer, and some lymphomas and leukemias, but show no potential for bowel, breast, or lung cancers. In addition the side effects can range from mild to life-threatening.

Q My aunt, who lives with us, has cancer. Is it infectious?

A No. There is no risk of catching cancer from a relative or a friend with the disease.

Q Do wounds ever become cancerous?

A Almost never—ulcers that have been present for many years can become cancerous, but this is very rare. An ordinary cut or graze never does. However, a lump in the skin that ulcerates should be seen by a doctor, because although ulcers rarely become cancerous, cancers often ulcerate.

Of all the medical conditions known, the one that creates the most fear in people today is cancer. But in many cases early diagnosis and continually improving forms of treatment can effectively control the disease.

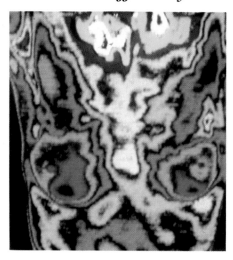

Thermography (heat X ray) is used in cancer detection—this shows no cancer.

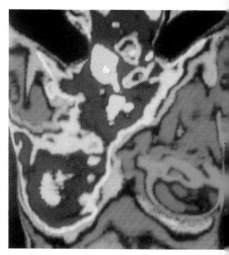

The red areas in this thermograph indicate the presence of cancer in the breast.

Cancer is the result of disordered and disorganized cell growth. This can only be fully understood by looking at what happens in normal cells.

The human body is made up of many different tissues—skin, lung, liver, etc., each of which are made up of millions of cells. These are all arranged in an orderly manner, each individual tissue having its own particular cellular structure. In addition, the appearance and shape of the cells of one organ differ from those of another. For example, a liver cell and skin cell look completely different.

In all tissues, cells are constantly being lost through general wear and tear, and these are replaced by a process of cell division. Occurring under strict control in normal tissues, so that exactly the right number of cells are produced to replace those that are lost, a cell will divide in half to create two new cells, each identical to the original. If the body is injured, the rate of cell production speeds up automatically until the injury is healed, and then it slows down again.

The cells of a cancer, however, divide and grow at their own speed and in an uncontrolled manner, and they will continue to do so indefinitely unless treatment is given. In time they increase in numbers until enough are present for the cancer to become visible as a growth.

In addition to growing too rapidly, cancer cells are unable to organize themselves properly, so the mass of tissue that forms does not resemble normal tissue.

A cancer obtains its nourishment from nearby, normal cells and serves no useful purpose for that person whatsoever.

Cancers are classified according to the cell from which they originated. Those that arise from cells in the surface membranes of the body (the epithelial tissues), like the skin and the lining of the lungs and gastrointestinal tract, are called carcinomas; those arising from structures deep inside the body, such as bone cartilage and muscle, are called sarcomas.

Carcinomas are much more common than sarcomas. This may be because the cells of the surface membranes need to divide more often in order to keep these membranes intact.

Benign and malignant tumors

Not all tumors are cancerous. Although tumor cells will grow at their own speed, tumors can be benign or malignant. Benign tumors tend to push aside normal tissues, but do not grow into them. Cells of a malignant tumor (a cancer), however, grow into the surrounding normal tissue, a process called invasion.

It is these clawlike processes of abnormal cells, permeating the normal tissues that are responsible for the name cancer —the crab—and its invasive properties. It is this that enables the cancer to spread, if unchecked, through the body.

The word *malignant* means "bad"; this can be contrasted with *benign*, meaning "harmless." Both accurately describe the outcome of the two types of tumor without treatment. A benign tumor can look almost like normal tissue when examined under the microscope. It behaves accordingly by respecting its neighbors. It also grows more slowly, and although usually harmless, it can be serious if it arises in an important part of the body, such as the lung. Benign tumors should be removed and surgery is nearly always curative.

Origin of cancer cells

Cancer cells develop from the body's own normal cells, and a single cancer cell is enough to start the growth of a tumor. However, the change from normal cell to cancer cell is a gradual one, taking place in a number of stages over several years. With each stage the cell becomes slightly more abnormal in appearance and slightly less responsive to the body's normal control mechanisms.

This process is usually unseen until a cancer develops, but in a few situations precancer can be recognized and treated. The best known of these is seen in the uterine cervix (neck of the womb), and this can be detected by a pap smear.

How cancer spreads

The abnormal growth is localized, at least at first, forming a mass in the location of the original cells. If surrounding tissue could be pushed aside, the cancer could be removed and the normal anatomy and function restored. This is not the case, however; the cancer usually invades the normal tissues very early. If these tissues are important, then life and health may be threatened.

The feature of cancer that accounts for most of its devastating effects is its ability to spread, or metastasize, from the original location to other regions of the body. This usually does not occur until the original collection of cells has grown to a fair size. The biological processes of metastasis are not fully understood, but good evidence exists that single cancer cells (or small clumps of them) break off

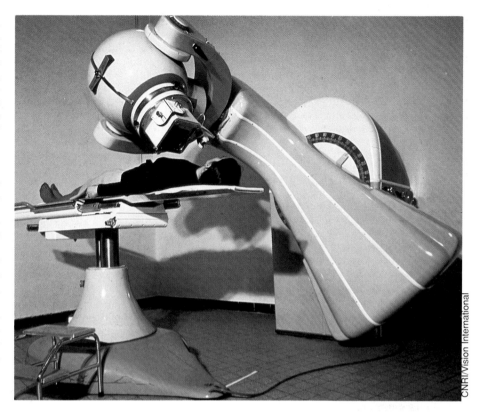

from the main cancer and are carried to other areas of the body by the blood or lymphatic system (see Lymphatic system).

Cancer cells carried by the blood are thought first to enter capillaries or very small veins or arteries. Once there they do not stop until they come to a place where the blood vessels divide to form channels so small that the cancer cells cannot easily get through. At such a point they may lodge and begin to grow, producing a new cancer mass much like the original. The first place this is likely to occur is the liver (for most cancers of the gastrointestinal tract) or the lungs (for most cancers starting elsewhere in the body), because these organs are the first places where blood from other organs is filtered through a network of minute blood vessels. Thus the lungs and liver are the most common sites of metastasis from blood-borne cancer cells. The cells can also, however, pass through the liver and lungs to lodge in other regions of the body—often in the bones or structures of the head and trunk, but also in other parts.

Normal lymph drainage begins in the peripheral lymphatic vessels, proceeding through a sequence of small structures called lymph nodes, and finally reaching one of the large central veins. These nodes, which serve as filters, contain many tiny channels through which the lymph and any cancer cells or other foreign matter must pass. Cancer cells that manage to pass through the lymph nodes

This patient is undergoing cobalt therapy, one of the newest methods used in the treatment of cancer. It acts by destroying the invading cancer cells.

and enter the bloodstream probably metastasize in the same way as cells that enter the blood directly.

Causes

Cancer is most common in late-middle and old age. Thanks to developments in sanitation and modern medicine, people are living longer, and this may contribute to the increasing frequency of cancer in the Western world.

Of course some cancers are associated with the Western way of life. Cancers due to smoking are still rare in the developing world but are becoming more common as industrial development takes place there and more people start to smoke.

The most common forms of the disease are lung, bowel, stomach, pancreas, and breast cancer. Despite developments in modern medicine, cancer is still responsible for a large number of deaths in the United States each year.

The most common cancers in children and young adults are leukemias (see Leukemia), sarcomas, and kidney cancer. Fortunately these cancers are rare, and their treatment has improved greatly in recent years. The cause of cancer is unknown, but two fundamental abnormalities are recognized. First, cancers are not subject to the normal influences that

Steps you can take to avoid cancer
- Stop smoking
- Drink in moderation
- Examine your breasts or testicles once a month for lumps
- Have a cervical smear done at least once a year
- Eat a balanced diet
- Avoid repeated sunburn if you have a fair complexion
- See your doctor if you develop persistent pain, bleeding, or a lump

Q My uncle has had radiotherapy once and has now been told he has to have a second treatment. Is this safe?

A Not if it is given to the same part of the body, unless it is a very small dose. The doctor will know how much that part of the body will tolerate and will only have advised a second course of treatment knowing it is safe. It is possible to give a full course of treatment to a different body part.

Q Can cancer ever be hereditary?

A Not usually. There are a few cancers that run in families, but these are rare and will be known to the families concerned. Only if cancer is particularly common in your family, is there any increased risk; if this is so, take better care of yourself, and report any persistent symptoms to your doctor.

Q I have been smoking up to 60 cigarettes a day and am worried about cancer. How many should I cut out to be safe?

A You should be worried! You do not say how many years you have been smoking, but it could well be that you have damaged your lungs irreversibly already— though this may not necessarily be cancerous. As far as cutting your consumption is concerned, the advice can be summed up in two words: stop altogether!

Q I have read that cancer is sometimes stress related. Also I have an aunt who literally willed herself to live against all odds. Is cancer a case of mind over matter?

A This is an interesting question, and there is no definite answer. There are cases, especially within families, where the fear of getting cancer when one person has become affected, seems to bring it on in others. So perhaps fear does act as a trigger. In the same way, sheer determination has been known to get an individual out of the trickiest situation, as your aunt's case seems to indicate. The answer is that no one really knows for sure.

control cell growth; second, the body will tolerate the presence of the cancer without rejecting it as a foreign invader. This makes them difficult to deal with.

Environmental factors, such as chemical pollution and exposure to radiation, are thought to lead to cancer, but there are several other factors that work together to the same end. The viral theory states that a cancer cell is infected by a virus (a tiny germ; see Viruses) that causes the cell to grow.

The immunological theory considers that abnormal cells are constantly being produced by the body but that these are destroyed by the body's defenses. For some unknown reason this defense system breaks down, and an abnormal cell survives to form a cancer.

The chemical theory relies on the knowledge that certain chemicals—tar, for example—will cause cancer when painted on the skin of laboratory animals.

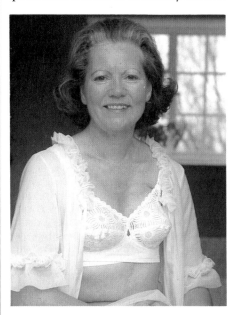

This woman suffered from cancer and had a mastectomy 22 years ago to remove her left breast. She now wears a prosthesis (artificial form of light synthetic material) under her bra.

These chemicals are irritants that may alter a cell's genetic structure and turn it into a cancer cell. Large numbers of experiments have identified chemicals that will cause cancer in animals; these are called carcinogens. A certain number have been identified, the best known being tobacco smoke. However, despite research, it has not yet been possible to identify carcinogens responsible for many of the common cancers.

Radiation is known to alter the genetic material of a cell—radiation from the atomic bomb dropped in Japan in 1945 is

thought to have caused cancers in the population, even years later. Since no single theory explains all the facts about cancer, it seems probable that it has many causes, some of which are still unknown.

Cancer screening

Cancer may be discovered because it causes symptoms that lead the patient to seek medical help, or it may be found by special screening examinations beforehand. The earlier a cancer is detected and treated, the higher the chance of a cure.

Much research has been done on developing screening examinations to detect cancer early. The greatest success has been the pap test to detect carcinoma in the cervix. The test is effective, quick, simple, and inexpensive. A few cells are scraped off the cervix, put on a microscope slide, dyed, and examined. Any cancerous cells may sometimes be destroyed without removing the uterus. If this is not possible, surgical removal of the uterus will cure the carcinoma and prevent cancer (see Pap smear).

Screening examinations of women without symptoms are also effective for the early detection of breast cancer, especially for women past the age of 50. A combination of physical examination, study of medical history, and mammography (a special kind of X-ray test; see Mammography)—all performed at one year intervals—can reduce mortality from breast cancer in this age group by at least one-third. Present methods do not seem to work as well for women under

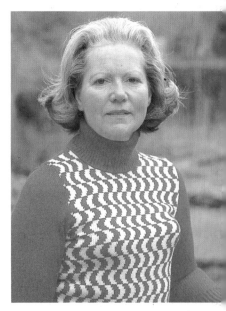

Here it is impossible to detect that she is wearing a prosthesis. So it is easy to see that a mastectomy does not have to mean the end of an attractive appearance and a full and enjoyable life.

Smoking and cancer

These statistics are based on a study of British doctors' smoking habits over a 20-year period. They show that the risk of getting lung cancer increases from 2.5 times that of a nonsmoker to 25 times as the number of cigarettes smoked per day increases.

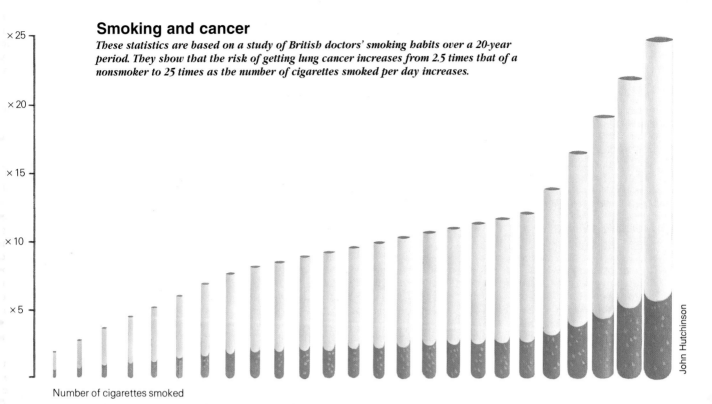

Number of cigarettes smoked

John Hutchinson

50, but regular screening is still recommended as early as 35 for women who are in groups known to be at especially high risk: those who have had a mother or sister with this kind of cancer and those who have already had breast cancer.

Two good methods exist for detecting cancer of the colon and rectum before symptoms occur: careful medical examination and tests for small amounts of blood in the feces.

Screening examinations have also been proposed for some other kinds of cancer, especially for persons known to be at high risk. It is currently felt, however, that extensive screening of the general population is not advisable because of the high costs of such tests, the low yield of unsuspected cancers, and the lack of documented improvement in survival. Some work has also been done on a "universal" cancer test to detect several (or even all) forms of cancer at once, but results thus far have been disappointing.

Diagnosis

It is no longer true that cancer is always fatal. There has been a vast improvement in the treatment of cancer in recent years, and many thousands of people are treated successfully. However, a small cancer is much easier to cure than a large one, so early diagnosis is vital and is helped by the prompt reporting of significant symptoms to the doctor. If the doctor suspects the possibility of cancer, he or she will refer the patient to a specialist.

The diagnosis will first be confirmed. This may initially involve X rays (such as a mammography in the case of breast cancer) and scanning tests to show the presence of a lump inside the body. A part of the tissue will then be examined under the microscope. This can be done either by biopsy or by cytological examination.

A biopsy is the surgical removal of a piece of the tumor, which is then sent to a pathologist to examine (see Biopsy). This will determine whether the suspected tissue is cancerous or not. Cytological examination is where body fluids, such as sputum or mucus from the uterine cervix, are studied specifically for cancer cells.

A thorough clinical examination is made, taking particular care to check the lymph nodes adjacent to the tumor. Simple blood tests are run to check liver and bone function and a chest X ray to look for evidence of spread into these sites. If the doctor is suspicious that cancer has spread to a particular part of the body, this area may also be scanned.

Various techniques are used. In isotope scanning, a very small amount of radioactive substance is injected into the body, and the blood then carries it to the suspected organ or area of tissue. If the tissue does contain a cancer, the cancer will take up a different amount of the isotope compared to the rest of the healthy tissue. The patient is then scanned with a special instrument that detects the radiation and the cancer can be seen. Many

organs of the body can be examined in this way, bone and liver scans being the most commonly performed.

After medical examinations have gathered detailed information about the type of cancer involved and the stage of its development, the doctor will, with the advice of cancer specialists known as oncologists, set a course of treatment. The techniques of cancer treatment are advancing and changing rapidly; it is sometimes difficult to understand which treatments are most likely to succeed in controlling the disease.

Surgery

Effective cancer surgery aims at removing all of the cancer from the patient. It usually involves removing the visible growth with a wide margin of surrounding normal tissue to make sure every cancer cell has been removed. In addition the surgeon will remove the draining lymph nodes and examine any adjacent structures. After removing the tumor, the surgeon will, where possible, reconstruct the patient's anatomy.

There are some circumstances in which surgery is carried out without investigating the patient first. When the patient is presented as an emergency case, surgery is performed both to diagnose and treat the patient. There are also some situations when a biopsy and a cancer operation are carried out under the same anesthetic. For example, it is common practice to biopsy a breast lump, examine the tissue, and then perform more extensive surgery if the lump is found to be malignant. Alternatively, a small biopsy may be taken in the surgeon's office and sent to the pathologist. This permits the patient to be aware of the diagnosis before the surgery is performed and to participate in making the decisions about proper therapy.

Radiotherapy

The aim of radiotherapy (see Radiotherapy) is to destroy the cancer with irradiation. Radiation damages the genetic material of cancer cells so that they are unable to divide. Unfortunately it also damages normal cells, but thanks to the body's remarkable ability to repair itself, large doses of radiation can be safely given—provided that it is given slowly enough.

Radiotherapy is given in special rooms with thick floors, walls, ceilings, and windows. Radiation leaks are thus prevented and the safety of the hospital staff insured. The patient lies on a special couch beneath the machine, and the machine is aimed at the tumor.

Before the treatment, the radiotherapist will have taken careful measurements of the position of the tumor to work out the best angle or combination of angles at which to set the machine. The staff then leaves the room before the machine is switched on. It is essential that the patient is in exactly the same position for every treatment. The treatment only lasts a few minutes and is painless—it is usually given daily for five to six weeks on an outpatient basis (see Outpatients).

Radiotherapy is not without side effects, but these can be kept to a minimum by careful medical supervision. Soreness of the skin is less of a problem today and is avoided by infrequent washing of the treatment area. Soothing creams are also given to the patient. Sickness and diarrhea are only problems when the abdomen is treated, and they can usually be controlled with drugs.

Loss of hair may occur if the head is treated, but hair usually regrows within six months, although the color and texture of it sometimes changes. Damage to other parts of the body is now rare, since the dosage that sensitive organs, such as kidneys and lungs, will tolerate is well known, and this dose is not exceeded. The treatment itself is painless.

Radiotherapy is used for localized tumors in addition to surgery. Some cancers of the head and neck can be controlled with radiotherapy without the need for surgery. In other situations radiotherapy can be given either before or after an operation to increase the chances of successful cure (as in cases of breast cancer).

In some circumstances it is possible to implant radioactive substances inside the cancer. These implants give a very large dose to the cancer itself with only a small dose to the surrounding normal tissue. This form of treatment is ideal, as the damage to normal tissues is kept to a minimum. Unfortunately it is only possible in accessible tumors, such as small cancers of the tongue and mouth and some that are gynecological in nature. Radiotherapy is also very good at relieving the symptoms, particularly the pain, associated with lung and bone cancers.

Cytotoxic chemotherapy

If a cancer is too widespread or metastases are present, it may not be possible to irradiate it completely or effectively. In this situation drug treatment is now available. The drugs used combine with and damage the genetic material of cells so that they cannot divide properly. The drugs were originally developed from mustard gas. Soldiers recovering from this form of poisoning were noticed to have low blood counts. It was quickly realized that the gas was interfering with the division of cells in the bone marrow, where blood is made.

Nitrogen mustard (the active drug in mustard gas) was therefore tried in cancer patients in an attempt to poison the cancer cells, and this proved successful. Treatment has now been greatly refined; many new and safer drugs have been discovered, and effective combinations of drugs have been developed. Unfortunately these drugs poison all dividing cells, hence the term *cytotoxic* (cell poison).

The best way to minimize the damage to normal cells is to give fewer, larger doses of cytotoxic drugs over a short period of time. There is then a gap of a few weeks (usually three) before the next course of treatment. This allows time for normal cells to recover.

The cells in the body that divide the fastest are the cells of the skin, gut, and bone marrow. The possible side effects of cytotoxic drugs include hair loss, nausea, and lowering of the blood count.

Hair loss occurs with a few of the cytotoxic drugs, but the hair regrows when treatment stops. The patient will be warned if hair loss is likely to be serious, and a wig may be provided. Nausea sometimes follows the injection of some

Symptoms of common cancers

Type	Symptoms
Breast cancer	Breast lump, bleeding from the nipple, indrawn nipple, change in the shape of the breast
Lung cancer	Persistent cough, spitting up blood, shortness of breath, chest pain, hoarseness
Cancer of the larynx	Persistent hoarseness, spitting up blood
Cancer of the esophagus (gullet)	Increased difficulty in swallowing, vomiting, loss of weight
Cancer of the stomach	Difficulty in swallowing, vomiting, bringing up blood, loss of weight, indigestion
Cancer of the bowel	Blood in the feces or from the rectum, a change of bowel habit—either constipation or diarrhea, or abdominal pain
Cancer of the bladder	Blood in the urine
Cancer of the prostate	Increased difficulty in passing urine, recurring urinary infections and back pain
Cancer of the uterus or cervix	If menstruating, bleeding in between periods; if postmenopausal, vaginal bleeding. Offensive vaginal discharge, lower abdominal pain
Cancer of the mouth and throat	Sore ulcer refuses to heal; pain in ear or ears; difficulty in chewing, swallowing; dentures increasingly do not fit
Leukemia	Tiredness, pallor, repeated infections, sore throat, bleeding from gums and nose, bruising
Skin cancer	Sore skin that will not heal and continually bleeds

This nine-year-old girl is suffering from acute lymphoblastic leukemia (a cancer of the blood). Treatment includes a two-year course of chemotherapy, which has caused her hair to fall out.

cytotoxic drugs but usually lasts only a few hours. Drugs that combat nausea can be prescribed. Alternatively, when it is expected to be severe, the patient is admitted to the hospital, and the treatment is given under sedation. However, this is rarely necessary.

The safe dosage for the various cytotoxic drugs is now known by the doctor, so serious depression of the blood count is now a much rarer occurrence than it used to be. However, the blood must be regularly tested both before and during such treatment.

Chemotherapy is not solely used for solid tissue tumors. It is also used to treat blood cancers, such as leukemia, because it has proved effective on bone marrow. Other cancers, like Hodgkin's disease, may respond better to chemotherapy than to extensive radiotherapy.

In some cases where there is an inclination to relapse after surgery and/or radiotherapy, chemotherapy is given even when there is no sign of cancer present. This is called adjuvant chemotherapy and is being tried in breast cancer and childhood cancers. Very encouraging results have been obtained, though it is still too early to advocate this kind of treatment for all cancer patients.

Hormone therapy

Hormones are chemical messengers that circulate in the blood to control the growth and metabolism of tissue. If cancer cells arise in a hormone-sensitive organ such as the breast, they may continue to recognize and respond to hormonal messages. If the patient is then given an inhibitory hormone—one that tells the cells to stop dividing—the cancer will stop growing. This type of treatment is sometimes used to manage breast and prostate cancers. In women, side effects such as hot flashes may result.

Combined treatment

Where more than one treatment is effective in treating a cancer, it makes sense to consider combining them in a planned, logical sequence of treatment. In some childhood tumors, surgery is followed by local radiotherapy and then one year of chemotherapy. The results are very encouraging.

In head and neck cancer, chemotherapy is followed by local radiotherapy, and then any part of the tumor remaining is removed surgically. Much research is now being carried out to determine the way

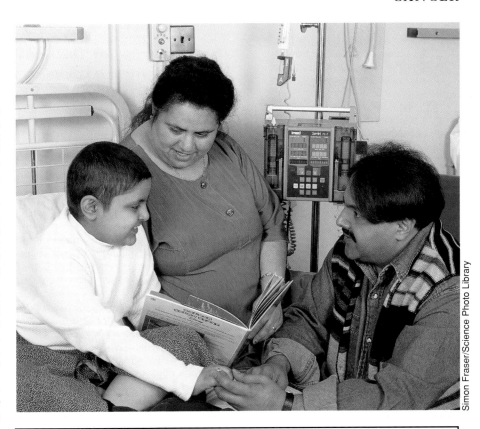

Simon Fraser/Science Photo Library

Differences between benign and malignant tumors		
Type of growth:	**Benign**	**Malignant**
	Pushes normal tissue aside	Invades normal tissue
Spread:	Slight	May form secondary growths
Structure:	Similar to normal growths	May be disorganized
Rate:	Slow	May be slow to rapid
Outcome:	Usually harmless	May be fatal if untreated
Treatment:	Surgery curative	Surgery alone may not be curative

of combining treatments of all the various cancers in order to make the best possible use of all of them.

Whole body irradiation and bone marrow transplantation

In recent years it has been possible to transplant bone marrow from one person to another. This very specialized procedure requires large doses of radiation to be given to the recipient of the graft beforehand—called whole body irradiation. At present this treatment is usually only used in rare forms of anemia and leukemia. In the future, however, it may be possible to treat other forms of cancer in this way.

Outlook

Many cancers can be successfully treated in their early stages. The importance of regular cancer screening must be emphasized so that early diagnosis and immediate treatment can take place. Any persistent, unexplained symptom must be reported to a doctor. Following a course of treatment, the patient is carefully monitored on an outpatient basis. Regular examinations of the original cancer site are made, and any new symptoms are investigated. For most forms of cancer, if the patient is alive and well five years later, then there is room for optimism. Advances in medical research are increasing the chances of surviving cancer.

Capillaries

Q I have recently developed some odd, purple patches on my skin. What can they be?

A The capillaries in the skin are normally supported by fibers of a stretchy substance called collagen, but as you get older, these fibers gradually become weaker and eventually collapse. Because the capillaries are then unsupported, they cave in—and this shows up as purple patches or lines. There are so many capillaries in the body that the loss of these few unsupported ones does not matter. The patches were once thought to be a sign of cancer, but this has now been proven to be totally untrue.

Q I have always bruised very easily. Does this mean I have weak capillaries?

A Yes. The walls of your capillaries could be more fragile than average, but this is nothing to worry about. Only if you get a crop of tiny bruises without any injury should you see a doctor, for these can be a sign that something is wrong with your blood.

Q Why does drinking make my face turn pink?

A Alcohol has the effect of dilating, or widening, the capillaries of the skin. The same effect can be brought about by hot drinks or exposing the skin to rapid temperature changes. If this happens very often, the capillaries can become permanently stretched. This shows up as a pinkness of the skin that does not die down. The best way to prevent this problem—which is most common in women over 30—is to avoid excessive alcohol and temperature changes.

Q Do all parts of the body have the same number of capillaries?

A No. Those parts of the body that need the most oxygen and food have the most capillaries. These include the kidneys, liver, heart, and the muscles involved in body movement. Supporting structures, such as tendons, have few capillaries.

The capillaries are the smallest blood vessels in the human body. They form a complex and vital network.

The capillaries form an extensive network of vessels between the arterial system (which takes the blood from the heart) and the venous system (which returns the blood to the heart). Each capillary measures only about eight-thousandths of a millimeter—only just wider than one single blood cell. The capillaries' job—one of the most essential in the human body—is to deliver oxygen and other vital substances to the cells and to collect the cells' waste products, which they do through their thin walls.

Structure

Capillaries are very simple structures whose walls consist of little more than a single layer of very thin, flattened cells called endothelial cells, which are connected together edge to edge. Each capillary consists of a very thin layer of tissue rolled up into a tube and surrounded by an equally thin membrane. All the capillary walls are thin enough to allow certain substances to pass in and out of the blood. The distribution of capillaries in the body is so rich that if all the structures of a person's body were removed except the capillaries, the person's individual shape would still be recognizable.

Capillaries are not all the same structure. Electron microscopy has shown that in different locations the capillaries may vary quite widely. Those in the kidneys, the lining of the intestines, the endocrine glands, and the pancreas, for instance, are perforated by tiny pores of widely differing size.

Those in the brain differ considerably from those in the rest of the body, especially in thickness. Their thicker walls provide what is called the blood-brain barrier. This is an effective obstruction to the passage of certain drugs and other substances from the blood to the brain cells and the cerebrospinal fluid (the fluid that surrounds the brain). This barrier offers protection for the brain against many potentially damaging substances commonly found in the blood, but it does have the disadvantage that it can interfere with treatment like antibiotics and other important drugs. Doses of antibiotics may have to be increased to many times those that are needed for infections elsewhere in the body.

Connecting link

As the heart pumps blood through the body, the blood goes first through the

Close-up of a capillary (right). Transfer of substances from blood to surrounding tissues happens in three ways (below)—water, food molecules, and hormones go through pores; oxygen and carbon dioxide are exchanged via walls; protein molecules are engulfed by capillary walls, then released outside.

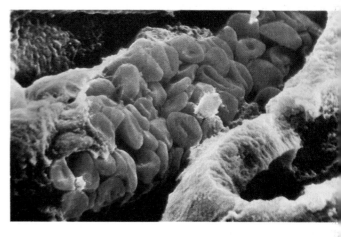

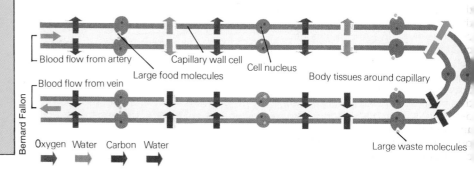

Blood flow from artery — Capillary wall cell — Large food molecules — Cell nucleus — Body tissues around capillary

Blood flow from vein

Oxygen Water Carbon Water Large waste molecules

Bernard Fallon

arteries. The arteries divide into branches called arterioles. The branches become smaller and smaller, and the smallest of them are called capillaries. In the capillaries the blood cells jostle along in single file, giving up oxygen, nutrients, and other substances, and taking in carbon dioxide and other waste products from the cells. When this process is finished, the blood needs to return to the heart. As this return journey starts, the capillaries join to form small veins that gradually grow larger as many branches join them.

Chosen route
When the body is resting, blood tends to flow through so-called preferential, or preferred, channels. These are capillaries that have become larger than average. But if extra oxygen is needed by any particular part of the body—for example, by the muscles during exercise or by the heart—blood flows through nearly all the capillaries in that area.

Capillary gaps
All capillaries have small gaps between the edges of the cells forming their walls. These gaps are very important. The pressure of the blood in the capillaries is very low, but it is highest at the arterial end of any capillary (the part through which blood enters the capillaries) and lowest at the venous end (the part through which blood leaves the capillaries). As a result of this, some of the watery part of the blood, but not the red cells or large protein molecules, passes out through the gaps and pores in the capillary walls at the arterial end. Most of this fluid passes back in through the walls at the venous end of the capillary.

Outside the capillaries, this fluid is called tissue fluid. It bathes the cells of the body, allowing diffusion of various important dissolved substances from the blood to the cells, and from the cells to the blood. This is how oxygen, nutrients, vitamins, minerals, hormones, and so on are able to get to the cells from the blood, and how waste products of cell metabolism are carried away from the cells to be disposed of via the bloodstream.

There is another important reason for the gaps in the capillary walls. Although these are too small to allow red blood cells to pass through, cells capable of changing their shape can do so. These cells are said to be ameboid, and they pass through the capillary wall gaps in a remarkable way. First the cell pushes a tiny finger through a gap. The substance of the cell then flows along this finger and expands outside the capillary. This process continues until the whole of the cell is outside. Cells of this kind belong to the immune system of the body and are called phagocytes. Their function is to combat infection, and millions of them pass through capillary walls at the site of any inflammation.

Sinusoids
There is one particular class of capillaries that differs from all other capillaries. These are called the sinusoids. The sinusoids are of wider caliber and are more irregular than other capillaries. But the most striking difference is in the number and size of the openings in their walls. The sinusoids in the liver have numerous, relatively large openings grouped so as to form sieve plates, which allow molecules below a certain size to pass through. Those in the spleen have long, slitlike openings in their walls that, unlike capillaries anywhere else in the body, allow whole blood to pass through into the surrounding space.

Regulating body temperature
In addition to the exchange of substances, the capillaries located in the skin play a special role—they help to regulate body temperature.

When the body is hot, the capillaries in the skin get wider, making it possible for a larger than usual volume of blood to reach the skin, where it can be cooled by the air outside the body. Capillaries widen and narrow passively as a result of changes in the pressure of the blood within them. This, in turn, is determined by the flow rate in the tiny arterioles supplying the capillaries. Arterioles have muscle fibers in their walls, which can tighten to narrow the vessels or relax to widen them. These muscles are involuntary—a person cannot control the way they work. Rather, they are under the control of the autonomic nervous system and the endocrine system.

Vulnerable skin capillaries
As they are very thin-walled, the capillaries can be easily damaged. Those most at risk are the capillaries in the skin. If the skin is cut, scratched, or otherwise injured or if it receives a hard blow, the capillaries release their blood. A bruise is the aftereffect of the capillary blood collecting in the skin.

Capillaries can be destroyed by burning, but they do have some ability to renew themselves. As a person grows older, or as the result of drinking excess alcohol over a long period, the capillaries may collapse, leaving purple patches or a network of reddish lines.

If the skin receives a heavy blow—in this case a kick from a horse—the capillaries in the skin's surface break and release their blood. This released blood causes the skin to discolor—the familiar bruise.

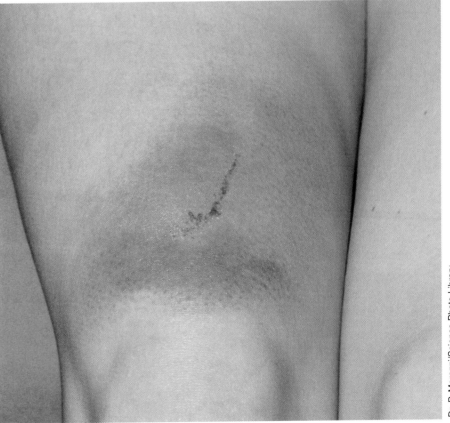

Cardiac massage

Q How much time should elapse after cardiac arrest before giving cardiac massage?

A Cardiac arrest is a medical emergency. If you check to see if there is a pulse rate and find none, you must begin resuscitation immediately. Lack of blood flow to the brain for three or four minutes usually results in brain damage. Although you might be able to get the heart beating again, the patient might die from the brain damage, or if he or she should live, there may be permanent mental impairment. If more than 10 minutes goes by before beginning resuscitation, the heart will be irreparably damaged.

Q What should be done if a person has a cardiac arrest while eating and their mouth is filled with food?

A Since cardiac massage and mouth-to-mouth resuscitation are given together, it is important that there is no obstruction to the airways while the latter is being performed. Therefore you must remove any food from the person's mouth and throat; the head should be sideways while you are doing this. Tilt the head back by pulling or pushing the jaw out, and move the tongue from the back of the throat. Close the nostrils with your fingers, and breathe into the patient's mouth. If the chest does not expand, you have either left some food in the throat or your technique is faulty.

Q If I saw someone collapse in the street, how would I know whether they had had a cardiac arrest?

A A sudden collapse does not necessarily indicate that a person has had a cardiac arrest; it could have happened for other reasons. However, there are a number of signs to look for. First establish if the person is conscious. If not, check to see if there is a pulse and if the person has stopped breathing. Look for any signs of the skin turning gray, and see if the pupils are dilated. If these signs are present and the person appears dead, start cardiac massage without delay.

Cardiac massage is one of the methods used to stimulate the heart into action when it has stopped beating. The technique will restore breathing and circulation and save a life if applied correctly.

Cardiac massage, or *cardiac compression*, is the name given to the first-aid technique used to stimulate blood flow from the heart by pressing on the patient's chest wall. External cardiac compression (ECC) is always given together with expired air resuscitation (the kiss of life): the two together are called cardiopulmonary resuscitation (CPR).

Cardiac compression is given in cases of cardiac arrest; when, because of a number of possible conditions, the normal rhythmic beating of the heart becomes disturbed, the contractions may stop. Cardiac arrest can be caused by a variety of factors: drowning, asphyxiation, hemorrhaging, electrocution, drug overdose, cardiac infarction (blocking of blood circulation), coronary air embolism (an air bubble in a vein that reaches the heart), or pulmonary embolism (an obstruction of the pulmonary artery by a blood clot).

Symptoms of heart failure

Although an electrocardiogram (ECG)—a test that shows the pattern of heartbeats on a graph—is needed to detect whether the heart has actually stopped, there are certain signs that indicate that the patient is experiencing cardiac arrest and circulatory failure. Around 6 to 12 seconds after the heart has stopped, the patient will lose consciousness. No pulse will be felt. Fifteen to 30 seconds after circulation has ceased, breathing will stop. The skin will turn gray, and the pupils will become dilated.

If these signs are present, resuscitation is urgently required to restart circulation and breathing. There is only a maximum of 10 minutes in which to do this. Within three or four minutes of the circulation ceasing, the heart will become damaged because of lack of oxygen. And although the heart may be restarted, the brain will suffer irreversible damage.

Blood flow

The principle of cardiac massage is that, by rhythmic compression of the chest wall (replacing the action of the heart muscle), blood flow will be generated in the carotid arteries (which supply blood to the brain) to resuscitate the brain.

What happens to the heart and to the blood flow during external compression is that, as the resuscitator squeezes down, blood is driven from the heart and from all the large vessels within the chest.

Backward flow of blood is prevented by valves at the point where the great veins of the head enter the chest.

The chest therefore can be thought of as a large sponge full of blood that is emptied by one massive squeezing motion, which is sustained for about half a second. At this point the aortic valve, which stands between the aorta (supplying blood to the whole body) and the left ventricle (the main pump from which the blood to the body comes), slams shut and prevents all the pumped blood from flowing backward into the heart. During relaxation, the sponge reexpands and blood runs back to fill the spaces formed. With the next squeeze of the sponge blood is further driven forward. The process is then repeated.

Performing cardiac compression

In case of cardiac arrest, heart massage should be started immediately. No special equipment is necessary, nor is the help of a doctor required.

Lie the patient on his or her back on a hard surface. Check to see if there is a carotid pulse by extending the head backward and feeling with all four fingers in the groove between the Adam's apple and the strap muscles of the neck. Allow yourself at least 10 seconds to be sure no pulse is present.

Move your hand down to the chest to the lower third part of the sternum (breastbone). Place your fingers at the point where the ribs join; there is often a small bone here called the xiphoid. Place the palm of your hand on this point, and then place the palm of your other hand immediately on top of it.

Press down; the movement should be rhythmical and regular, at a rate of 60 times a minute. Make sure that you keep your hand on the chest wall and that you press only in the mid-line between the nipples. For an adult you should apply the full weight of your body. Children and babies require a much lower pressure; use one hand or a thumb.

When one person is combining cardiac compression with expired air resuscitation, he or she should blow in two breaths during every 15 heart compressions, but no pause in the heart cycle should be allowed for a breath to be given. If two people are working together, one of them should blow in one breath for every five compressions that the other gives. Although in adults the ideal rate is 60 beats per minute at an uninterrupted rhythm, in children this rate should be speeded up. Infants and children up to five years old should be squeezed at about 100 beats per minute, those between the ages of five and ten at about 80 beats per minute. Older children should receive compressions at 60 beats per minute (as for adults).

The carotid pulse should be checked every two minutes during the massage to see if there has been a return of pulse. Once this occurs, you can stop cardiac compression. Usually the heartbeat will be restored within a few minutes. The patient will begin to breathe again, the gray hue of the skin will disappear, and the dilated pupils will return to normal.

Dangers
There is no danger of starting up an irregular heart rhythm or stopping the heart, but overenthusiastic compression of the chest may damage the soft organs that lie under the lower parts of the ribs. The result is that there may be a rupture of the liver, stomach, or spleen. On occasion ribs may be broken, but this is one of the hazards of performing a life-saving procedure. Generally if the hands are placed in the correct position and heart compression is done properly, no damage should be done. It is important that a squeezing action with adequate force should depress the sternum only by 1 to 2 in (2.5 to 5 cm).

First aid for cardiac arrest

FIRST AID

Heart massage combined with the "kiss of life"

First loosen the unconscious patient's clothing. Check that the airways are clear by running your finger inside the patient's mouth. Check the carotid pulse, which is stronger than the one at the wrist. If you are in doubt, put your head to the patient's chest, slightly to the left of the lower end of the breastbone, and you will be able to hear if there is any heartbeat. Remember that seconds matter, so start immediately—don't wait for the ambulance. Finding the carotid pulse is a technique best learned before it is needed. Practice on yourself by placing your fingers and thumb each side of your neck, below the jaw, until you feel it. Tilt your head back slightly and place your fingers between your Adam's apple and strap-neck muscles.

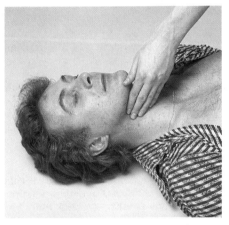

Lie the patient on his or her back on a hard surface. Feel the carotid pulse by extending the head backward and feeling with your fingers between the Adam's apple and the strap muscles of the neck.

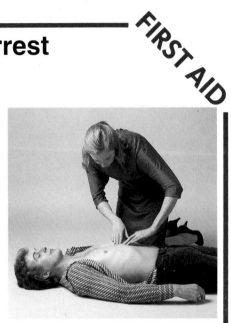

Establish the position of the heart by running your fingers down the chest to the lower third part of the breastbone. Place your fingers at the point where the ribs join (you may be able to feel a small bone here).

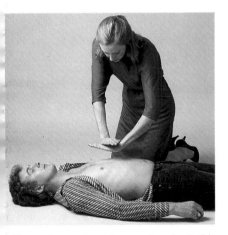

Place the palm of your hand at this point, and then place the palm of your other hand on top of it. Press vertically downward, rhythmically, 60 times a minute.

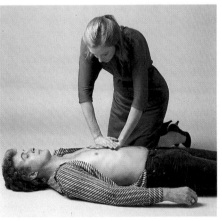

Make sure you keep your hand on the chest wall, pressing only on the line midway between the nipples. Apply the full weight of your body for an adult—use less pressure on a baby or child.

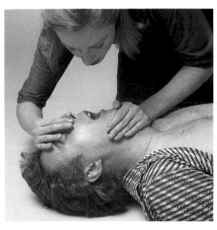

Mouth-to-mouth resuscitation has to be given simultaneously. If possible, someone else should do this. A breath should be blown in after every fifth heart compression.

Brian Nash

Carpal tunnel syndrome

Q I am expecting my first baby soon and have developed weakness and tingling in the first two fingers and thumb of my right hand together with pain in my forearm. My obstetrician says it will get better by itself after the baby is born, but what is causing it, and is my obstetrician right?

A You are suffering from carpal tunnel syndrome, brought on by the swelling—or edema—that is common in pregnancy. It tends to be worse in the mornings when you first get up, and it is the classic reason why pregnant women drop things. This symptom can be a warning that you have the sort of edema that may indicate a more serious condition of pregnancy called preeclampsia. If you have none of the other symptoms of preeclampsia, such as raised blood pressure or traces of protein in your urine, both of which will be checked for at your prenatal visits, there is no need to worry. The symptoms nearly always disappear completely soon after delivery.

Q Does carpal tunnel syndrome only affect the hands?

A Similar conditions can occur if the nerves at your ankle or elbow become trapped, though both these conditions are far less common than carpal tunnel syndrome. A trapped nerve at the ankle is called tarsal tunnel syndrome. The principal symptom is intermittent burning or numbness in the sole or toes of the affected foot, sometimes also spreading up the calf, that gets worse as the day goes on. If you have a trapped nerve at the elbow, you may feel tingling or numbness in your little and ring fingers.

Q Does carpal tunnel syndrome affect men and women equally?

A This common condition does occur in both men and women, but the majority of sufferers are middle-aged women.

Our hands are extremely sensitive and capable of a wide range of movements, but in carpal tunnel syndrome both sensitivity and movement are reduced as the flow of messages between the brain and the hand is restricted.

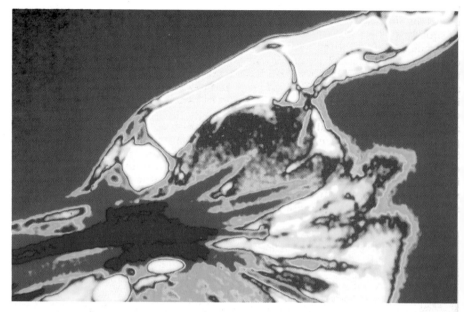

This color magnetic resonance imaging (MRI) scan shows the hand of a person suffering from carpal tunnel syndrome. The bones of the thumb (top) show white, the tendons and ligaments (left) show blue and pink. The carpal tunnel lies under these ligaments.

The hands are among the most sensitive parts of the human body, especially the surfaces of the fingertips. They are also extremely powerful and versatile, being capable of performing a very wide range of movements, many of them extremely intricate. A number of nerves carry signals between the brain and the hands, controlling how the hands move and how they feel. It is the pinching of one of these nerves—the median nerve—as it passes through the wrist that leads to the condition called carpal tunnel syndrome.

Structure of the hand and wrist

The hands and wrists are made up of a number of small bones and joints. Each hand contains five bones in the palm, called the metacarpals. One end of four of these bones is joined to a finger, which consists of three bones, or phalanges, with a joint between each. The end of the fifth metacarpal bone is joined to the thumb, with two phalanges and a single joint. The hands are joined to the bones of the forearms—the radius and the ulna—by the wrists.

Each wrist is made up of eight separate bones called carpals. They are arranged in two rows and are bound together by about 20 ligaments and tendons (see Tendons). The bumpy wrist bone that is visible through the surface

of the skin is one of the carpals. The tendons and the median nerve that supply the hand are enclosed in a tough membrane that prevents the tendons from stretching the skin when the hand is flexed (pulled forward). The wrist bones above and the membrane below form a tunnel called the carpal tunnel. Because this passageway is narrow and rigid, if the tissues inside it swell for any reason, they crush the nerve and tendons, pressing them against the bones.

Symptoms and causes

Carpal tunnel syndrome may affect one or both of the hands and usually begins with a sensation of numbness, especially in the thumb and the next two and a half fingers, as the median nerve is crushed. This is followed by pins and needles, the unpleasant, tingling feeling that occurs as the crushed nerve recovers and sensation returns to the hand and fingers. The forearm and the thumb are often also very painful. The pain is generally worse at night and may be bad enough to wake a person from a deep sleep. The reason why the condition should be more painful at night is not clear, but if this is the case, hanging the hand over the side of the bed and rubbing or shaking it can sometimes help to lessen the pain.

The symptoms may be brought on by overusing the hands for intricate work, such as sewing or knitting, or by activities that involve strenuous or repeated use of the wrists, such as playing tennis or squash.

Carpal tunnel syndrome can also be caused by other medical conditions, including diabetes, rheumatoid arthritis, and an underactive thyroid gland. An individual may also develop the syndrome if he or she fractures the wrist and causes some internal damage that puts pressure on the median nerve. Some women also find that they develop the syndrome during pregnancy, but in this case it nearly always disappears shortly after the birth, when the swelling that caused it also disappears.

In some people the condition is particularly severe, and it causes permanent numbness and weakness of the thumb and one or more of the fingers.

Treatment

Most people who suffer from carpal tunnel syndrome do not need any specific treatment. The symptoms gradually ease of their own accord as soon as the swelling or pressure affecting the nerve is reduced, for example, by stopping a strenuous or repetitive activity. Wearing a splint on the affected wrist at night may help to ease the pain. It is advisable not to take up a similar form of activity, even when the symptoms have disappeared, without consulting a doctor.

In some cases the doctor may advise treatment with drugs. Diuretic drugs will reduce the amount of fluid in the swollen tissues, and an injection of an anti-inflammatory drug into the wrist joint can help to reduce inflammation, both of which will reduce the pressure

on the nerve. In individuals whose carpal tunnel syndrome is caused by diabetes, rheumatoid arthritis, or an underactive thyroid gland, good control of these diseases can improve the carpal tunnel syndrome.

If the syndrome is particularly persistent, or if it recurs at frequent intervals or causes severe pain, it can be permanently cured by surgery to reduce the pressure on the nerve. This may involve cutting through the tough membrane to create more space for the nerve. Sometimes some of the swollen or damaged tissue is removed at the same time. The procedure is usually highly successful, and the symptoms disappear immediately. It leaves only a small scar on the inside of the wrist that soon fades to become insignificant.

Sports that involve strenuous or repeated use of the wrists can sometimes lead to carpal tunnel syndrome. In such cases stopping the activity may be necessary.

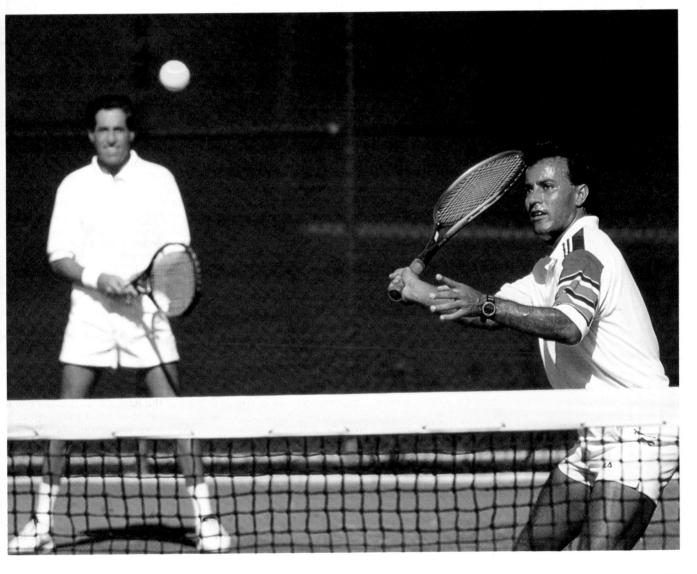